Psilocybin Therapy

Dr. JJ Pursell, ND, LAc.

PSILOCYBIN THERAPY

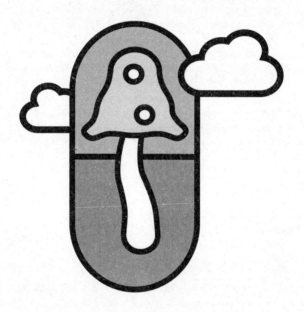

UNDERSTANDING HOW TO USE NATURE'S PSYCHEDELICS FOR MENTAL HEALTH

Timber Press
Portland, Oregon

Timber Press
Workman Publishing
Hachette Book Group, Inc.
1290 Avenue of the Americas
New York, New York 10104
timberpress.com

Timber Press is an imprint of Workman Publishing, a division of Hachette Book Group, Inc. The Timber Press name and logo are registered trademarks of Hachette Book Group, Inc.

Text design by Sarah Crumb
Jacket design by Vincent James

The publisher is not responsible for websites (or their content) that are not owned by the publisher. The Hachette Speakers Bureau provides a wide range of authors for speaking events. To find out more, go to hachettespeakersbureau.com or email hachettespeakers@hbgusa.com.

ISBN: 9-781-64326-200-0

A catalog record for this book is available from the Library of Congress.

To all of those who came before
and honored this medicine,
I thank you.

....

Contents

Preface 9

Acknowledgments 12

Introduction 14

....

CHAPTER 1. **The Wonders of Fungi** 21

CHAPTER 2. **Why People Use Psilocybin** 33

CHAPTER 3. **History of Psilocybin** 53

CHAPTER 4. **The Effects of Psilocybin on the Brain** 77

CHAPTER 5. **The Role of a Facilitator** 85

CHAPTER 6. **The Session** 106

CHAPTER 7. **Integration** 127

CHAPTER 8. **Welcome to Your Shadow** 135

CHAPTER 9. **Microdosing** 147

CHAPTER 10. **Medical Considerations with Psilocybin** 163

CHAPTER 11. **Preparing for a Psilocybin Session** 173

CHAPTER 12. **Respect and Ethics** 183

....

Other Psychedelics 191

Psilocybin Retreats and Costs 195

Psychedelic Music Playlists 198

Psychedelic Harm Support 199

How to Become a Facilitator 200

Psychedelic Therapy Training Programs 202

Glossary 205

Notes 207

Bibliography 212

Index 223

Preface

WHEN I WAS FIRST PRESENTED with the opportunity to write this book, I dove in headfirst and began writing down everything I already knew about the subject and what I thought would be best for a beginner's guide. I wrote starter sections on cultural history, modern advancements, research, editorial bits, and so much more. But as with any book, the further you go down the rabbit hole, the more things begin to shift and morph. For me, this happened about eight weeks into the project. I gave myself a pause and truly asked myself, "Who am I to write this book?" I'm definitely no Bill Richards, María Sabina, or Kilindi Iyi. Nor does my background reflect the professional longevity with the subject of Janis Phelps, founder and director of the CIIS Center for Psychedelic Therapies and Research. Both James Fadiman and Ralph Metzner have already composed excellent texts on the purpose and complexities of a psychedelic journey. As I wrote, I also really struggled with presenting a decolonized telling of psilocybin history, and I definitely did not want to fill these pages with a retelling of the same story. I seriously questioned what I could bring to the table, particularly at this crucial juncture when psychedelic medicine is returning to the mainstream medical model—albeit early in its journey.

My foray into psychedelics began over thirty years ago. Many people have experiences with psychedelics in their teenage and college years, often in group or social environments. That is how most of my experimentation with psychedelics in my teenage years went. A few of us would take psychedelics together and either go to a large house party, go camping, or hang out at one of our homes. Despite the Reagan-era DARE messaging, I had never personally experienced or witnessed another person losing their mind while on psychedelics. My experiences at this time were based on the notion that psychedelics were "party" drugs, something you took on a Friday night to have a wild and crazy time—and most of my experiences were just that. Long nights with highs and lows, riding the roller coaster of psychedelics. The highs were filled with explosive laughter and the ability to feel deeply connected to my friends, and the lows often involved the unprocessed emotions of our lives. These lows might have led to tears or fear or anger because we were young adults doing our best to process the burdens of our lives.

But those early years evoked something in addition to the endless cascades of those teenage nights. After about an hour, as the psilocybin took effect, it would evoke thoughts, feelings, and new ideas—ideas that I grew more and more curious about. Often these feelings would connect me to something I had been missing, craving, or even grieving. The best way to describe what I was connecting to was that I was connecting to *me*. Through all the overthinking and superficial consumption of teenage life, I would find and connect with myself, which at the time was quite radical. To find a time and space where I didn't question or reject every aspect of myself was magical and so relieving! The depth of this connection filled my heart and soul with what I had longed for and had been searching for externally in my life—connection and, more specifically, connection to myself and the world around me.

Having these inner experiences in conjunction with the external ones with my friends became a duality. I was taking psychedelics (LSD and psilocybin) for both pleasure and so I could take deep dives into my inner self/soul. Both aspects offered me great insights, but the greatest of these was the ability to remember that I am a person, someone of value with love in my heart. As a young person, having a tool to better understand yourself in relation to the world is invaluable. At the time, these psychedelic experiences decreased my depression and anxiety and helped me succeed in ways I never thought I would.

As I've gotten older, psilocybin (and, to a lesser extent, LSD) has become a tool for my well-being. I find great value in its support of a positive mental outlook. Despite coming from a place of privilege (as a white, middle-class, cis female), I've had a moderate amount of mental health struggles in my life. Thankfully, I have learned to turn to psychedelics to provide clarity and to help maintain a healthy frame of mind.

Psychedelics have an extensive history of use outside of the United States, as well as a reputation marred by decades of false and politically motivated stories. With the recent return of psychedelics to both clinical research and the Western therapy model, there will be struggles to deconstruct the biases against these valuable medicines. For some people, under medical guidance, there is no doubt of the benefits of psilocybin. While we move into this emerging medical paradigm, hopefully our society can begin to shift away from the negative connotations that have plagued psychedelics since the 1960s.

In recent years, my professional journey with psychedelics has shifted once again. I live in Oregon, the first state to legalize the medical use of psilocybin. Through witnessing the bureaucratic process of implementing a legal system around psilocybin use and learning from many of the leaders in the field, this is not necessarily going to be an easy road. But the education I received at the California Institute of Integral Studies, my experiences as a facilitator of psilocybin sessions, and the incredible psychedelic community give me hope that together we will continue to grow, advocate, and educate about the potential benefits awaiting many of those who are suffering.

As I share my research, the history, and select testimonies from those who have experienced psilocybin, I hope you come to view this powerful entheogen with fresh eyes and an open heart. For those that suffer, the potential benefits are innumerable.

Through the writing of this book, I have often been humbled by what I've learned about myself. As it turns out, though, I have a lot to say about this subject that I think you'll find valuable. As a regular person, struggling in perhaps some of the same ways you are, I hope you find this book easy to read, relatable, and helpful in your journey toward self-discovery and healing.

Acknowledgments

I HAVE A LOT OF PEOPLE to thank for this book. First and foremost, all of those who came before me who have held the sacredness of the magic mushroom. Without you, I would never have been able to put my thoughts and words down on the page. It is because of them and the mushrooms themselves that I've been led to where I am now. Thanks must also be given to all of my teachers—who have been working with this medicine, with the knowledge of its ability to ease suffering—and to their never-waning belief that someday we'd be able to offer it to those in need in a safe and legal way.

To my original editor and trusted ally, Stacee Lawrence, for giving me the chance to write the magical mushroom book (not a culinary one) that had been brewing in my mind for quite some time. Your wit, intelligence, and skills are unparalleled. And to Will McKay, thank you for jumping in and helping me see this to completion.

The idea for this book began brewing when I was called to join a mushroom cultivation class in Jamaica taught by Darren Springer (a.k.a. Darren Le Baron). It was that class—and later a friendship with Darren—that allowed me room to stretch my knowledge in new and exciting ways. Darren, thank you for keeping me grounded in the medicine, reminding me of the value of connection, and teaching me to always be open to the suggestion.

A big thank you to all my colleagues at the California Institute of Integral Studies, as well as the professors including Mary Cosimano, Bill Richards, David Presti, Tony Bossis, Ben Sessa, Anthony Black, Jen Matthews, Chanda Williams, and Kwasi Adusei who all impacted me with their teachings and words. I must also thank Janis Phelps, the director of the Center for Psychedelic Therapy and Research, as she was a huge inspiration through her leadership and integrity of the profession.

Mel Torrefranca, we've never met, but it was your playlist on YouTube that kept the writing zone flowing and I'm so grateful for your creations!

Lastly, as always, to my big and amazing family, thank you for the unwavering support in all that I do. Cordelia, thank you, thank you, thank you for bringing laughter into my life every day and for making me laugh at myself and the crazy world we live in. Tommy, thank you for loving the wonder of the mushrooms as much as I do. Brian, your consistent love and support are a pillar in our life together. And while I love all our animals, sweet little Maui came into our lives at the beginning of this project and has remained in my lap throughout the duration.

Introduction

I'VE ALWAYS BEEN ATTRACTED to doors, especially when traveling—picture the ornate doors of Turkey, Morocco, and Portugal. There is an almost irresistible urge to open every intricately carved door I see, for something so beautifully unique must contain something equally beautiful on the other side. It is this feeling that drives the human experience: the curiosity of what is on the other side, the hope that we'll find nirvana or perhaps the peace and understanding that we search for. I feel the same when I meet new people. They show me their unique and exquisite exterior as I marvel with curiosity, wondering what gloriousness must be on the inside. Psilocybin allows us to open the door to ourselves and see the incredible beauty on the other side.

I am fascinated with the natural world. While I consider myself a free spirit, there is a side of me that needs structure, organization, and scientific evidence. Because of this—and in conjunction with my background in biochemistry and medicine—it has been important to me to try to decode the possible physical, mental, and emotional benefits of using psilocybin as a medicinal healing agent. As I discuss psychedelics within a therapeutic medical model, I will also focus on my background as a non-lineage-holder of the psilocybin tradition. I am a Western clinically trained psychedelic facilitator. While my background is colorful, it is my personal relationship and the Western model that I primarily draw my experience from.

Historians of psychedelics in the United States typically speak of R. Gordon Wasson, who wrote "Seeking the Magic Mushroom" for *Life* magazine in 1957; Timothy Leary, an American psychologist and strong advocate for the use of psychedelic drugs; and Albert Hofmann, the Swiss chemist who first synthesized lysergic acid diethylamide, or LSD. While many Western researchers made important clinical contributions to the field of psychedelic research, the long Mesoamerican/Mexica history of psilocybin use, as well as that in other regions such as Africa and Greece, is rarely discussed. I hope to elevate this cultural history back to its proper place before moving into the subsequent Western history of psilocybin that was only made possible due to our predecessors.

We are currently in a period of reclaiming psychedelics, with individual states decriminalizing psilocybin and initiating measures to use it as medical treatment, with a primary focus on mental health and addiction. When looking back through the history of psychedelics in the United States, however, it is difficult to not feel frustrated with the imposed limitations and setbacks of clinical research on these substances, because the many who suffer with mental health and addictions could have been benefiting from these medicines for decades.

Psychedelics—also known as psychoactive agents, hallucinogens, and entheogens—were commonly researched in the United States throughout the 1950s, 1960s, and early 1970s. Before psychedelic use took a highly politicized turn, international clinicians, scientists, and researchers met yearly at multiple conferences. Laboratories around the world conducted research, writing more than 1000 peer-reviewed articles supporting the use of psychedelics for mental health and as a positive support for psychotherapy.

So, what caused the dormancy of American psychedelic research between 1977 and 1999? An unfortunate combination of politics, societal unrest, sensationalism, stigma, and stereotyping. The contrived, amplified messages against psychedelics impacted both our governmental systems and our local communities, creating divisions between those who accept and reject these substances. (The War on Drugs is discussed in Chapter 3.) But despite these divisions, the underlying truth is that clinicians and researchers had already delivered scientific proof of psychedelic's therapeutic efficacy, with research outcomes repeatedly

Entheogens

....

An entheogen is a psychoactive substance that induces the feeling of God, or cosmic spirit, within oneself or a feeling that we are all connected, one of self-love, acceptance, and belief. Carl A. P. Ruck, a classics professor at Boston University, coined the term *entheogen* in 1973, which he discusses in his book *Mushrooms, Myth & Mithras: The Drug Cult That Civilized Europe*. Ruck's introduction of the term was his attempt to create a word that could describe the psychedelic experience. Psychiatrist Humphry Osmond and others also recognized the need for a word to explain the thoughts and feelings that one experiences while on psychoactive substances. This is how the term *psychedelic* was born. Unfortunately, the term was tarnished through the belief that these substances caused delirium, criminality, and abuse.

The psychedelic state can be compared to the state of mystic consciousness, an idea originating from the Greeks, which is a state of being in which one feels the presence of something greater than oneself. Throughout history, monks, Sufis, poets, religious leaders, and others have reported their connection to a "greater source." What they experience, see, and feel has led to philosophies and historical outcomes still embraced today.

Psilocybin is considered an entheogen because it often creates an experience similar to mystic consciousness. When ingested, psilocybin can shift one's consciousness and perception and allow individuals to experience something of spiritual significance.

demonstrating a positive change in participant's beliefs, mental health, and well-being after their use.

An important aspect of clinical research is dosage and outcome. Psilocybin can be used in various dosages, depending on the intention and treatment goal. Moderate doses—between 2 and 3 grams of dried mushrooms—are commonly used in clinical trials for more profound outcomes. Traditionally, larger doses have been used in many cultures around the world for rites of passage and other ceremonies. Microdosing is the ingestion of very small doses (microdoses) that do not elicit a psychedelic response. I'll discuss microdosing in Chapter 8, but it is fast becoming a mainstream tool to spark creativity, remain balanced within oneself, alleviate depression, and support connection with others.

One of the greatest benefits of psilocybin use is the potential to open oneself up to new insights and perceptions, to go in search of the self-love and acceptance reported in clinical findings. According to a 2020 study conducted by the National Institutes of Mental Health, major depressive disorder affects approximately 17.3 million Americans, and over 21 percent of Americans report having had at least one or more depressive episodes in their life. Nineteen percent of Americans have been diagnosed with anxiety, with many more likely going undiagnosed. To alleviate suffering and support positive communities, mental health needs to be a priority. Endless studies have been performed on the benefits and side effects of medications commonly used for depression and anxiety, and it is clear that we need to pivot. At the very least, psilocybin's clinical history and outcomes deserve to be considered on the short list of possible treatments for those dealing with these issues.

Various groups are currently involved in different stages of clinical research on psilocybin and MDMA (3,4-methylenedioxy-methamphetamine, commonly known as ecstasy, molly, or mandy), with Johns Hopkins University and the Multidisciplinary Association for Psychedelic Studies (MAPS) leading the way. An article published in the *Journal of the American Medical Association* in November 2020 reported that treatment for depression with psilocybin was even more successful than projected.[1] The report's author Alan K. Davis noted, "The magnitude of the effect we saw was about four times larger than what clinical trials have shown for traditional antidepressants on the market." Although psilocybin is still classified as a Schedule I drug, this wave of research has not demonstrated that psilocybin's mechanism of action has an addictive or dependence tendency—it does not light up the reward centers of the brain like addictive substances.

Psilocybin and other psychedelics are now starting to be integrated into both the mainstream and medical model. Honestly, I'm somewhat incredulous at how far the needle has moved in just the last three years. If you have begun to test the waters with self-research in the psilocybin space, you probably know how quickly you can become inundated with websites, social media links, classes, and conferences. It can be challenging to navigate, so wherever your research or practice leads you, please consider the following questions:

What drives the information/person you are following? It is important that capitalist gain is not the driving force.

What sort of training does the person have? Training is important, because psychedelic harm is a very real thing. Training can take a lot of different forms, both academically and culturally.

How is cultural bias and implicit bias being addressed in the information you are finding? With the long history and negative impacts of psychedelics in the Western world, we need to ensure that the principles of practice and information being presented are inclusive and accurate.

My aim in this book is to provide you with a solid foundational overview of the current psilocybin and psychedelic terrain. I want to empower your curiosity and give you a safe place to explore. Throughout the chapters you will find the duality of scientist and spiritualist that I spoke of previously. I would not do the subject justice by sharing just one or the other with you.

In closing, I share several testimonies, which often offer the most profound contemplation regarding the use of psilocybin. While every experience is different, testimonies provide a glimpse into what an altered state or psychedelic experience can really feel like.

"I didn't feel anything mystical or out-of-body. It was more the opposite. It's like the most body you will ever be."

"Once I was past the darkness, I began to feel an increasing feeling of peace and connectedness. . . . An intense feeling of love and joy emanated from all over my body, and I can't imagine feeling any happier. I knew that the worries of everyday life were meaningless and that all that mattered were my connections with the wonderful people who are my family and friends."

"I was reveling in the undeniable feelings of infinite love. I said [to myself], 'I am love, and all I ever want to be is love.' I repeated this several times and was overwhelmed with the intensity of the love. I was aware of tears flooding my eyes at this point. All the other goals in life seemed completely stupid. . . . There were so many incredible moments; so many intimate and intense moments of self-acceptance, self-love, and self-honoring, which is paramount. I went into my trip thinking I would uncover some sad truths about me not being a good person or uncovering something ugly about myself, and the opposite was true. It allowed me to give myself a long, much-needed inner hug. The most important takeaway is that the things I discovered were always within me, truths I'd already known, but I'd pushed away. Maybe I wasn't willing to face them, maybe I didn't feel that my intuition was strong enough . . . . Whatever the reason, it became clear that everything I need to know is inside of me. Those truths uncovered in a totally different state of consciousness allowed me to observe them without judgment and accept them for what they are. I learned about my purpose and, with ongoing processing, am trying to understand how to integrate what I learned into my life."

CHAPTER 1

The Wonders of Fungi

ONE OF MY FAVORITE WRITERS, Wendell Berry, once said that herbalism—the study of plant medicine—is based on relationships. Here in the Pacific Northwest, we are blessed with nature that inspires the mind and promotes peace in the heart. Even if you aren't the outdoorsy adventurous type, the natural beauty that surrounds this region is hard to ignore. Yes, we have endless months of rain during winter and spring, but as early as January we are starting to see signs of spring and by mid-March cherry blossoms fill the horizons. We have what seems like an endless palette of greens and terrain that ranges from the mountains to the sea. We also have loads and loads of mycelia, the branched vegetative filaments of the fungi. When I first heard this word, I became fascinated. Not just because it is a cool word to say, but because of the role mycelia play in sustaining forests, plants, soil invertebrates, and entire ecosystems. When we speak of relationships, mycelia and the fungi that come from them connect us all.

I've decided to begin this book where I believe it should begin, with a thorough discussion of the therapeutic medicine, psilocybin. The modern history of medicine mostly originates in laboratories and pharmaceutical companies, but *Psilocybe*—the genus of psychedelic fungi commonly used to enhance mental health—comes from nature. Having the knowledge and understanding of what you put into your body, where it comes from, and how it will affect you is, I believe, part of the healing process. Words like *magic mushrooms* and *psychedelics* have a lot of stigma attached to them, and we are going to tease that out in the next chapter. For now, let's focus on the facts. Psilocybin has been used for centuries by cultures around the world, and it has been researched for more than seventy years in the United States. It seems we are on the precipice of legalizing psilocybin use for the treatment of mental health issues, addiction, and post-traumatic stress disorder (PTSD), as well as for self-enlightenment. Oregon has already graduated the first cohort of legal psilocybin facilitators, and many states are close behind. So let's start with where this medicine originates.

Fungi are a group of spore-producing organisms that feed on organic matter and include molds, yeasts, mushrooms, and toadstools. And they've been around for a long time, my friend, predating humans by millions of years. Scientists have discovered 90-million-year-old specimens in amber, and fossilized fungi have been unearthed that date back 420 million years. The next time you go for a walk in nature, turn over an old log or gently lift up decaying fall foliage and you'll see fungal mycelia in action.

What you'll see are thin, white filaments that vary in size. These filaments are called hyphae, and they are the first step in mycelium development. Hyphae result from spore germination; once hyphae are established, they utilize the forest to nourish themselves and grow. They start eating whatever they can around them, becoming the tiny composters of the forest. And they grow fast. My son and I recorded hyphae growth in the forest near our home: they went from 0.2 to 1 inch in just two days! Soon enough, the threads reach the mycelium phase. Depending on their maturity, mycelia may be extremely small or grow into larger branched networks spreading in multiple directions, networks so big that they can expand across the entire floor of large forests. These once-microscopic organisms penetrate the soil to grow and connect everything that grows around them. Their system is referred to as the mycorrhizal network, which stems from two Greek words: *myco* meaning "fungi" and *rhiza* meaning "root." From a botanical and biological perspective, these networks connect everything. Yes, everything! The networks connect to other networks, to all the surrounding plants and

Did Mushrooms Come from Outer Space?

....

Theories abound that fungal spores arrived on Earth from outer space. Read up on panspermia and American ethnobotanist Terence McKenna's belief that mushrooms came to Earth from meteorites that had spores on them. Researcher Janine Fröhlich-Nowoisky and her colleagues have reported that many fungi are capable of global dispersal via airborne spores. We'll get into psychedelic mushroom nomenclature later, but *Inocybe*, one of the genera which contain psilocybin, is capable of long-distance, transoceanic dispersal and *Psilocybe*, the genus to which "magic mushrooms" belong, also likely has this capacity.

I love to consider the possibilities that the evolution of humankind was the result of spores from a galaxy far, far away landing on Earth. Or the idea that human brain evolution was influenced by eating psilocybin mushrooms. As my teacher and mycologist colleague Darren Springer (Darren Le Baron) says, "We're all mushrooms having a human experience."

trees—basically everything within the ecosystem. Mycorrhizal networks were dubbed the "woodwide web" by Suzanne Simard, as it is through mycelia that trees communicate. When we talk of plant communication, mycelia are the mother lode of switchboard operators, the communication network of the Earth.

Functionally, mycorrhizal networks transport water, carbon, nitrogen, and many other minerals to mature trees, saplings, shrubs, low-lying forest plants, and soil invertebrates. Just like humans have basic nutrient needs, plants require a proper balance of the aforementioned things to be healthy and survive. But illness and disease are present in the environments of every living organism, plants included, and this is where it gets interesting.

When you walk through the woods, have you ever noticed there are a few trees that stand out from the rest? They are usually the tallest or the healthiest looking ones with the thickest trunks. Once you start looking, it can be easy to spot the big "mother trees" (a term coined by ecologist Suzanne Simard). They are the largest, oldest, yet healthiest trees dispersed throughout the forest. These mother trees have the biggest mycorrhizal networks at their base, and they use those network in surprising ways. With their giant roots, they can pull up water and other nutrients from deep inside the Earth, which helps maintain their life and health. But mother trees don't just pull up water and nutrients for themselves—they also pull it up to disperse to the surrounding vegetation utilizing the mycorrhizal network.

The idea that trees communicate in various ways is not a new concept; Suzanne Simard and Peter Wohlleben are two scientists who have written extensively on the subject. To give an example of what this may look like, think of a sapling that isn't receiving enough sunlight to photosynthesize the nutrients it needs to survive. A mother tree close by can detect distress signals through the mycorrhizal network, just like a parent who hears a baby crying, and respond with lifesaving measures by sharing necessary nutrients.

But this relationship isn't one-sided. Mother trees have large mycorrhizal networks at their base and utilize them to sustain life, but the mycelia also benefit by receiving a bountiful supply of photosynthate, the end products of photosynthesis. Fungal hyphae and mycelia cannot photosynthesize and therefore cannot produce sugars and other vital nutrients. They must explore the soil, and it is this hunt for sustenance where we see fungi's important role in the forest decomposition and regeneration cycle. It is hyphae that break down the plant matter around them so that microbes can decay the materials back into their elemental forms and upcycle their nutrients back into the ecosystem.

So, how does all of this relate to psilocybin? Spores. Mushrooms are the fruiting bodies of mycelia—the flower of the plant, so to speak.

Keep in mind that not all mycelia produce fruiting bodies, but all fruiting bodies come from mycelia. When a mycelium fruits, it produces a mushroom, and mushrooms have an abundance of spores. Part of the life cycle of the mushroom is to release its reproductive spores, which can spread far and wide. (There are some amazing videos of this eruptive action on YouTube, but be forewarned that you can lose serious amounts of time once you start watching!) The spores float on the air (or water) to a new resting place and get to work, immediately sending out hyphae in search of food. The hyphae turn into mycelia and quickly grow so that 1 cubic inch of soil can contain enough mycelia to stretch 8 miles. In fact, the Pacific Northwest is home to the Humongous Fungus, a single mycelia network that covers almost 4 square miles in the Malheur National Forest.

Psychedelic Mushrooms, *Psilocybe cubensis*

I know you're ready for the deep dive into how psilocybin works therapeutically, but stay with me for just a little longer. As a naturopathic physician with a specialty in herbal medicine, I strongly believe in the power of nature. Naturopaths recognize the value of our natural world in assisting the healing process. Not only do we utilize substances that originate in nature we also incorporate a healthy natural environment as a foundational factor in human health. Psilocybin is a valuable medicine that comes from the Earth, and it's valuable to have some perspective on how its origins play a role in your healing process.

Therapeutic mushrooms are a specific genus of fungi called *Psilocybe*. There are more than 200 species within this genus, but for much of our discussion I'll focus on *Psilocybe cubensis*, commonly called "magic mushrooms." Most *Psilocybe* species live in humid subtropical forests, but they can also be found growing in some surprising environments, including in open fields, on decaying wood, on the edge of railroad tracks and parking lots, and—much to my delight—in the compost and mulch I spread all over my garden last year. The mycologist Paul

Stamets believes that *Psilocybe* species have a special affinity for environmentally disturbed areas, such as those that have been affected by floods, landslides, and volcanic eruptions. He explains that mycelia can easily move throughout the flow of debris, allowing new mycorrhizal networks to form. From this perspective, you can almost imagine mushrooms as a type of healer of the Earth, working to knit it back together and transport nutrients and other compounds to areas where they are needed.

Psilocybe cubensis, the most common variety found growing in North America, contains psilocybin and psilocin, the two alkaloids predominantly responsible for the psychedelic action in a mushroom trip/journey/session/experience.* In herbal medicine, we can identify a botanical as an action based on which chemical constituents it contains. Plants can contain a myriad of chemical compounds that perform many different actions. Each constituent, when isolated, can be classified by its action—whether it stimulates, sedates, nourishes, or detoxifies.

Plants and fungi contain many different constituents that help them develop, thrive, and survive. In addition to alkaloids, other examples you might be familiar with are tannins or flavonoids. Tannins are the constituents that can make wine taste and feel "dry" in your mouth. Flavonoids, on the other hand, have been shown to have a direct correlation to brain cognition. Researchers identified the individual constituents of many plants and predicted how they will affect the human body. Is it a perfect science? No, but having some consistent foundational knowledge is helpful.

In the case of *Psilocybe*, researchers have determined that the main constituents that create the psychedelic experience are the alkaloids psilocybin and psilocin. Keep in mind, however, that we are still early

---

* In this book I'll focus on the term *session*, as that is one of the commonly used terms in clinical trials and the medical model. I've chosen to avoid the word *trip*, as it has negative connotations remnant of the War on Drugs, and the term *journey*, which can be triggering for some.

in our scientific understanding of these fungi, so other constituents may also play important roles. Alkaloids can produce a wide range of reactions in the human body, but what is more interesting to me are the effects of *Psilocybe* when used as a whole. I want to better understand how all the mushroom's constituents work together to produce a psychedelic experience. We know that once a constituent is isolated from the whole, it often is diminished in action, so why not consider this principle with psilocybin? Some believe the secondary alkaloids baeocystin and norbaeocystin also contribute to the things we think and feel while in a session. I believe it is important to broaden the horizons of psilocybin understanding. As we move into a medical model of psilocybin use, it is being debated whether we should use the whole *Psilocybe* mushroom (in tea form, as a capsule, or ingested whole) or isolate these main alkaloids from the fungi and create a synthetic, pharmaceutical-grade capsule. As both options are available and in common use, when it comes to dosage it's important to understand that synthetic psilocybin is generally discussed in much smaller amounts (milligrams) than dried, whole mushrooms (grams).

In the study of herbalism, learning the concept of herbal energetics—how different constituents work together within the plant organism—is key to understanding how to use it to heal the body. Plants are dynamic living things, just like humans. Much like plants, humans have all sorts of checks and balances and a multitude of systems in our bodies that maintain our survival. As a doctor, I look through this lens when evaluating a person's health. Isolating symptoms or health patterns is rarely helpful when working with my patients. Doing so only creates the idea that symptoms can appear out of the blue, which in my clinical opinion is rarely the case outside of overt trauma. Evaluating the entire person is an important aspect of proper health care. The same goes for botanical medicine. I believe that the whole plant has much more to offer than one isolated constituent.

In pharmaceutical preparations, one isolate or one constituent is extracted to make a patented medicine. This was the case with psilocybin when it was marketed by Sandoz as Indocybin for basic psychopharmacological and therapeutic clinical research in the 1950s. Constituents were isolated, produced, packaged, and sold. While pinpointing a constituent's action is surely helpful, I am persistently questioning: If we don't use the whole plant, what other potential therapeutics are we missing out on? And which of those may have helped reduce a side effect?

Various *Psilocybe cubensis* Strains

Psilocybe cubensis is a naturally occurring species. But thanks to cultivation of this common psychedelic mushroom, which began in the 1970s, there are now hundreds of strains available. A strain is a subgroup within a species that has a particular morphology or chemical profile. All species are genetically distinct, so strains within a species have the same genetic code but some genes are more active than others. These variations can produce slight differences in how they look or feel or the actions they have on those who ingest them.[1] I mention this so you won't get confused when someone starts talking about Golden Teacher or White Albino, which are simply two different strains of *Psilocybe cubensis*.

In the wild, *Psilocybe cubensis* grows naturally all over the world. There are approximately twenty species of *Psilocybe* in Asia, fifteen in Australia, twenty-two in the United States and Canada, fifty-five in Mexico, forty in Central and South America,[2] six in Africa, and twelve in Europe. But after R. Gordon Wasson introduced Americans and Canadians to the magic mushroom through his article in *Life*, people took it upon themselves to learn how to cultivate these prized mushrooms—and it is a lot easier than you might think.

Unlike plant hybridization, in which two genetically distinct parent plants are crossbred to produce a hybrid, new mushroom strains are often the result of random genetic mutations. For example, if I cultivate an Albino A+ strain and end up with a flush—a group of fruiting bodies—twice the size that they normally should be, it is most likely the result of a random mutation. (This is not a bad thing, by the way.) Or let's say I'm cultivating Golden Teacher, which is normally brown on top, but the flush turns out to be all white (albino). This is another random mutation. By choosing the healthiest mushrooms from each life cycle, these random mutations can be selected and cloned for several generations to create a new strain in a process known as isolation.[3] New strains, such as Pink Buffalo, Amazon, and PF Classic, are then introduced into society.

So which strain is best? Just like asking a room full of herbalists which herb is best for a head cold, a group of mushroom cultivators will give you a lot of different answers. Most cultivators list the strains they grow with specific qualitative effects next to each given strain. These can include something like the following:

User: good for beginner

Effects: mild hallucinations, euphoric feelings, moderate visuals

Whether cultivating or wild-crafting—collecting from the wild (please don't do this without both knowledge and experience)—plants and mushrooms, energetics contribute to the final product. We know a person's energy can be measured and plants can communicate—read *The Secret Life of Plants* by Peter Tompkins and Christopher Bird for more. Therefore, it is easy to imagine that our energy affects the plants we grow. In the Mazatec culture of Mexico, they wild-craft mushrooms in a strict ritualist way, protecting the positive energy they believe lives within the fungi. Any tainting of that energy before ingestion will transfer into the participant. When I learned of this practice, it made me think of my own medicine-making days. I was fiercely protective of the medicine we made at my herb shoppe. Sometimes I would need to request that a staff member take the day off due to personal upsets that were affecting them. Practicing meditation or ritual to be able to uphold positive healing vibrations throughout the medicine-making process

Amanita: The Other Psychoactive Mushroom

....

You might recognize *Amanita* as the *Alice in Wonderland* mushroom. In the United States we think of them as a dangerous and poisonous mushroom, but in places such as northern Europe, *Amanita* mushrooms are considered a delicacy when prepared properly. Research has also begun regarding their psychoactive properties and potential uses for improving both mental and physical health. But before you run out to harvest one, please do your research and speak with an experienced mycologist.

is important. Just like herbalists, many curanderas—female leaders, typically within Hispanic communities, who have unique knowledge with regard to health and healing—believe each species of mushroom has its own power and that power can be translated into the exact lessons needed by the participant ingesting it. This power is demonstrated through the various experiences one has during a session. For instance, there may be more or less visuals, hallucinations, release of emotions, or euphoria.

Cultures that do not place a spiritual essence within the mushroom are more likely to believe that these differences in experience are related to variations among *Psilocybe* strains. In my personal opinion, however, the set and setting (which I discuss in Chapter 6) and your mindset going in have a greater impact on your experience than the strain you take. Yes, there are some strains that can consistently create experiences of intense visuals or specific sensations, but I feel that your intention and the preparation beforehand have the greatest influence on your experience.

Summary

When we begin considering psilobyin we can ponder many things, including whether mushrooms really did come from outer space or the role they had in human evolution. And when you consider all the different types of mushrooms, their active expulsion of spores, and their ability to travel incredible distances, as well as their varying colors and sizes and that some can even glow in the dark—it does make you wonder. But one thing is for sure, fungi have an incredible ability to grow and disperse worldwide. Thankfully, at some point along the way, the lives of humans intertwined with mushrooms, intentionally or accidentally. Understanding this relationship between humans and the experience the mushrooms provide has both intrinsic and extrinsic value to our well-being. Learning about what psychedelics are, how they affect us, and their potential usefulness in healing is the terrain we will now start exploring.

CHAPTER 2

Why People Use Psilocybin

AT THIS POINT IN THIS BOOK you may be asking, "Who around me is using psilocybin, and should I?" Maybe you've read the *New York Times* articles spotlighting moms who microdose and psilocybin sessions for the terminally ill. Perhaps you watched a Netflix documentary on the topic. Or maybe you've picked up this book simply out of curiosity. The reasons someone may decide to consider psilocybin therapy can be as extensive and as varied as the shades of a sunset. Some use psilocybin to lift them from repetitive depression or heal from traumatic life events. Others may see it as a thread of hope to find something within themselves that brings peace and joy. Psilocybin can be used to pursue connections with others or ourselves or for a deeper understanding of life in general. We may not even be able to vocalize why we want to try it, just that we feel guided to do so. There is often something within us wanting and reaching for something *more*, although the identity of that more is very subjective: more understanding, more knowledge, more love, more enlightenment, more healing, more experience, and so on.

Some reasons to participate in psilocybin therapy are more obvious than others. Attempting to resolve trauma or coming to terms with death are two examples. But just because you don't fall into one category or another doesn't mean psilocybin therapy isn't for you. Many of us are simply trying to dig deeper into ourselves and the life around us. You don't need to have a pinpointed intention for psilocybin therapy, but the more thought you put into it beforehand, the more you typically will get out of it.

I like to offer the Hindu philosophy of the Purushartha as a starting point when considering questions of why someone might like to try psilocybin. Below I'll get to specific reasons, but the Purushartha, or the four aims of human life, can be a helpful tool to help identify a more specific reason for therapy.* In general terms, the Purusharthas are the objects of human pursuit, working within a system to better understand ourselves, those around us, and the greater cosmos, which is similar to what psilocybin does. The first aim, Dharma, is for increased personal understanding. This includes a deeper understanding of self and can include the healing of trauma through self-reflection. When we better understand ourselves, we are true to our moral compass and can live the authentic values of who we are. You may be struggling with certain parts of yourself and wish to focus on that during your psilocybin session. Another area you might lean into during a session is the second aim, Artha. This aim reflects one's duty in life, gaining insight into how to help others, the world, and ourselves. In modern times we can refer to this as how we make money and our core values surrounding that. By diving into this aim, we can learn more about what motivates, scares, limits, or calls to us. With new insight into ourselves, we can pursue our career paths with an eye toward the greater good. The third aim, Kama, is for pleasure and enjoyment. Yes, it is okay to consider psilocybin therapy for pleasure. Sometimes we can lose the joy in our lives and not fully understand why. With the intention to experience joy in your psilocybin therapy, you can potentially open yourself up to bring in happiness. And the last aim, Moksha, is for transcendence or to experience a level of enlightenment. This is the aim that helps to better understand death and the dying process. As we'll discuss later, mystic experiences were one of the primary areas of focus in psychedelic research in the 1960s.

---

* Although I do not subscribe to any one religion, I do find value in various aspects of all different kinds of religious and spiritual practices, which help me better understand myself and the world around me.

Only Delinquents and Hippies

....

Many of you—if not the majority—may feel uncomfortable when we talk about using psychedelics or, specifically, magic mushrooms. This could be due to a programmed response based on negative societal messaging, growing up in the DARE era, or simply because they are illegal. Currently, the recreational use of psilocybin is illegal in the United States, with Oregon being the only state to have legalized its therapeutic use. Because of these uncomfortable responses, the medical model has transitioned away from words such as *trip, tripping, magic*, and *shrooms*. We refer to the mushroom by its Latin name, *Psilocybe*, and the active constituent psilocybin, which instigate less judgment than when viewed through the "magic mushroom" lens.

Because I live in a bit of a psilocybin bubble, I was curious how programmed the general public still was regarding psilocybin. When I asked a focus group who had never tried psilocybin why one might choose to do so, the themes were consistent: "Why would I want to do that?" "You'll lose your mind if you do that." "You'll lose all control." "Only delinquents and hippies use psychedelics." These responses were pretty much aligned with the messaging that the War on Drugs began over fifty years ago, but I was still slightly surprised by their prevalence today.

Our political and media outlets have done an excellent job of convincing the populace that psychedelics are dangerous and that under no circumstances would anyone of civility use them. The message has been reissued and reinforced throughout many decades, making psychedelic use taboo and frightening. However, the curious or experienced user realizes that this messaging is far removed from the truth.

When we decide to participate in psilocybin therapy, looking at these four areas can be helpful. However, sometimes these reasons are not clear or are locked away in our subconscious. As a result, it can feel confusing or difficult to vocalize why you wish to try psilocybin. But as a wise facilitator once told me at the beginning of a session we were about to do together, trying to have at least one reason will create room for more interpersonal work. I hadn't put in enough consideration for this particular session, and when I arrived I simply stated that I was open to whatever was supposed to happen. After a brief conversation about this, I understood her perspective. Remaining open to whatever was supposed to come up, without having an inkling of intention, can prevent you from going deep and opening the door for intentional healing. Contemplating the Purusharthas is one starting point, a tool that might help you better understand your reason for going into a session.

One of the greatest reasons why Americans have tried psilocybin over the last century was to find connection. In essence, psilocybin connects you to you. I know that seems rudimentary and reflects Timothy Leary's 1960s directive to "turn on, tune in, drop out," but that's what it does. Psilocybin enables you to see, think, and feel the truth of who you are and has a way of doing so that is predominantly gentle and reassuring. It allows you to explore the big questions of your mind, often leading you to a place of epiphany. These aha moments are the clutch of psilocybin. They allow you to integrate new meaning and understanding into your life—typically from a place of peace and calm. (In transparency, some psilocybin experiences can be challenging—I'll examine this more in later chapters.)

Spiritual enlightenment is another common reason to take part in a psilocybin session. Spirituality can be defined as the quality of being concerned with the human spirit or soul as opposed to material or physical things. In an attempt to find more or find spirituality, we focus on what is inside ourselves instead of what is outside of us. Psilocybin can give you the ability to plug in to yourself, to connect in a new way, and often allows you to better understand your beliefs.

But what does it mean exactly to connect with yourself or have a spiritual experience? Many books and articles on psilocybin talk about the guided transition from a normal mental state into a psychedelic state and how amazing it is. They describe this flowy, rainbow-filled, floating-on-a-cloud experience. There are accounts of wild geometric patterns and the ability to feel or hear colors. They talk a lot about a feeling of unity and self-love—even I will mention this. But what I want to emphasize is that there is no way to *know* what you will experience or how you will feel the first time you try psilocybin. It's honestly akin to childbirth. You can read every book out there, watch videos, take classes, and talk to other parents, but until you have the experience yourself, you just don't really know what it is.

I think Simon G. Powell says it best in *Magic Mushroom Explorer: Psilocybin and the Awakening Earth*: psilocybin amplifies the contents of the psyche, raising unconscious material into conscious awareness. For a first-time user, this can be a bit intense. It may feel chaotic and confusing. Sometimes there is so much noise it can be difficult to relax and wade the waters of the experience. When your brain begins to recognize yourself and the world in a new way, it can be challenging. But if you've prepared for the session and you have tools to navigate the tricky spots, the experience can be life-changing.

In honesty, asking the question "Why do people take psychedelics?" is like asking "What flavor of ice cream do you like?" to a hundred different people. There will be many different answers. But in the United States in the twenty-first century, the reasons are mainly geared toward improving mental health. This has been the focus of most of the clinical trials on psilocybin and is where we have the most data to determine psilocybin's benefits. One unfounded rumor regarding psilocybin therapy is that its use can lead to the *development* of mental health conditions and increased suicidal behavior. However, a 2015 study of mental health patients and their outcomes found no significant association between lifetime use of psychedelics and increased mental health treatment or suicidal thoughts, plans, or attempts.[1]

Psilocybin in the Hospice Setting

You may be familiar with research studies on the use of psilocybin with terminally ill cancer patients. In 2000, Johns Hopkins University was the first institution to receive regulatory approval in the United States to conduct psilocybin trials in a hospice setting. The researchers reported that treatment with psilocybin under psychologically supported conditions significantly relieved existential anxiety and depression in people with life-threatening cancer diagnoses. Michael Pollan's book *This Is Your Mind on Plants* and his article "The Trip Treatment," published in the *New Yorker*, have brought to our attention the value of this research.

Lessening anxiety surrounding death and creating opportunities to better understand our lives in conjunction with their endings are two examples of how psilocybin can help in these contexts. But it goes so much deeper than that. Patients who were involved in the Johns Hopkins studies experienced an incredible connection to themselves and the actual dying process. Most of those who had experienced extreme anxiety and fear of dying were relieved of those feelings after just one session and were able to live their remaining days with joy and peace. One of the first terminally ill participants in a Canadian psilocybin study said, "Magic mushrooms allowed me to calm the worries in my head, allowing my body to use my energy for healing instead and process the remaining fears in a supportive environment."[2] Data collected in similar studies show patients experiencing decreased anxiety and increases in feeling purpose in life, spirituality, and death transcendence.

Almost all the terminally ill patients who participated in this research had similar outcomes. What was commonly described before the psilocybin treatment as fear, anxiety, and hopelessness was replaced with peace and a sense of understanding. Life became much more enjoyable after the psilocybin dose, as the fear of dying went away and was replaced by feelings of unity and love. For humans, one of the hardest aspects of living is understanding and accepting that we will die. These studies and other reported experiences suggest that the use of psilocybin unlocks an ability to better understand what we are and how we are connected to the greater cosmos. With clinical findings such as these, making psilocybin accessible to patients in hospice settings would surely be of great benefit.

Let me now introduce you to a key figure in modern hospice, Dr. Cicely Saunders. Born in England in 1918, Saunders would later become the founder of St. Christopher's Hospice and the mother of the hospice care movement. After pursuing a career in nursing, she went on to earn a degree in social work, which she applied in the hospital setting, looking in on patients to ensure their well-being. Saunders's work went beyond the basic physical needs of the patient to also include friendship, which she began to view as an integral aspect of a hospice setting.

Early in her social work, she met a young Polish patient named David Tasma. He was only forty at the time and had no family or friends, and he was dying of cancer. The relationship that grew between them was pivotal in the manifestation of Saunders's future work. Out of this work and their conversations, she came to the realization that those who are dying needed everything that we could give of the mind—every skill, every understanding—but also what she called "the friendship of heart." She understood that you must provide physical and emotional care to support terminally ill patients, and she underscored the importance of the patient's ability to say yes to death. She believed that the human body has an innate wisdom of its own, and if the patient can manage to say yes to the ending of life, a transformation occurs. This transition to acceptance can be empowering, giving the person a sense of agency.

Coming to terms with death is one of our greatest challenges as humans. We have not been guided properly, and as a result we tend to hold fear in our hearts regarding the inevitable. As researchers at Johns Hopkins have demonstrated, the use of psilocybin has helped many patients find peace and understanding in the dying process. If we combine the potential of psilocybin with Saunders's foundational emphasis on spiritual and psychological care for hospice patients, I believe we have immense potential to alleviate anxiety and suffering surrounding death.

The Case of Chrissy

Chrissy was a woman in her fifties, diagnosed with stage 4 breast cancer with metastases in her lungs, who participated in a study of psilocybin-assisted psychotherapy.[3] She was a self-described atheist who was employed full-time as an administrative supervisor in the health care industry. She had never been married or had children, and she lived alone. She had personal experience using both psilocybin and LSD and received a diagnosis of generalized anxiety disorder upon screening.

Chrissy said that she knew she was beginning to experience the psilocybin effects when she could "see music," something she described as beautiful, comforting, and amazing. She remembered being surrounded by the cosmos, spirits, and light and hearing words inside her head in a voice different from her own, saying "We are here all together," a phrase she interpreted as welcoming her into this psilocybin-induced state. She describes a part of her experience: "I was seeing these kinds of stone faces, and they were beautiful, and they would kind of come to dust, and then they would come back up, and then they would come back to dust, so I kind of think of that as like, that's the nature of life. . . . It rises and falls; that's the normal way it is."

Chrissy experienced strong themes of unity and connection during this session, saying, "I felt like I could reach out to anybody and connect with them." At one point, Chrissy saw a Ferris wheel, which she interpreted as a circle in which "life comes from death and death comes from life." She experienced her own birth and explained, "I remember breathing, feeling my breathing, and then kind of feeling that I was coming up against a membrane of some sort. Then at some point, I came through it, and that was just amazing." She spoke about feeling pain in her abdomen and experienced this as her "umbilical cord to the universe," saying, "This was where my life would be drained from me someday and I would surrender willingly when my time came." Though Chrissy experienced a sense of being at peace with death, she went on to explain that she "chose to live" and that the experience helped her reach this decision.

After using psilocybin, Chrissy experienced significantly decreased anxiety, depression, death anxiety, hopelessness, and demoralization and increased purpose in life, spirituality, and death transcendence. Chrissy said, "At one point I asked, 'Is there going to be a cure for cancer?' [It] doesn't matter. We're all going to die—doesn't change it. That was my answer." When asked later whether her religious or spiritual beliefs had changed since her psilocybin session, she noted that the experience had "brought my beliefs to life, made them real, something tangible and true—it made my beliefs more than something to think about, really something to lean on and look forward to."

Promoting Mental Health

In the United States, psilocybin clinical research began in the 1950s and has had persistently positive findings. The focus continues to be within the mental health arena, treating anxiety, depression, addiction, PTSD, and negative thought patterns. For anyone who has experienced mental health issues, myself included, we can wholeheartedly say that there is very little we wouldn't do for relief. Studies performed by Johns Hopkins University showed that treatment with psilocybin relieved major depressive disorder symptoms in adults for up to a month. A follow-up study of those same participants showed that the substantial antidepressant effects of psilocybin-assisted therapy, given with supportive psychotherapy, may last at least a year for some patients.[4]

Psilocybin is often used in conjunction with psychotherapy to deepen patients' relationships with themselves and their personal struggles. This practice supports and potentially accelerates the healing process and the ability to understand what one might be struggling with. Many therapists have stated that *just one* psilocybin treatment is like accomplishing years of talk therapy. What they mean is that psilocybin has the potential to open us up to a new level of understanding and truths in a single session. In essence, it can catapult your mental/emotional self forward. This can be great as long as you have a qualified therapist to guide you through the integration process. As I'll speak about at great length in Chapter 7, for the beginner, integration is an essential part of any psychedelic self-discovery journey.

Attempting to process, release, and heal from traumatic events is another common session focus. Sexual abuse, childhood abuse, PTSD, and addiction are all examples of trauma that can inhibit a person from living a joyful life. *Acid Test: LSD, Ecstasy, and the Power to Heal* by Tom Shroder provides an inside look at the personal transformation of trauma survivors as they went through psychedelic therapy.

A team at Imperial College London, led by Robin Carhart-Harris, ran a trial with twelve participants, all diagnosed with treatment-resistant depression.[5] The study included two treatments with a 10 mg dose of synthetic psilocybin, followed a week later by a 25 mg dose. After nine weeks, nearly half of the participants reported that their depression had reduced by roughly 50 percent. As Michael, one participant in the study reported, "I became a different person. . . . I couldn't wait to get dressed, get into the outside world, see people. I was supremely confident—more like I was when I was younger, before the depression started and got to its worst."

Treating PTSD in Veterans

Psilocybin studies have provided hope for veterans with PTSD, depression, and anxiety. Polls have shown that 80 percent of veterans believe that the public does not understand them. Returning to civilian life can be debilitating for many veterans, and having no one who understands what they are going through often leads to mental health struggles. Psilocybin works to alleviate those struggles as a serotonin agonist—an agonist is a substance that promotes a biological response. Serotonin is a neurotransmitter thought to regulate anxiety, happiness, and mood. Before psilocybin clinical trials, veteran participants reported having crippling anxiety that made daily living almost unbearable. Combine this with the potential onslaught of mental anguish experienced due to flashbacks and an inability to contribute to their families, their communities, or themselves and we end up with a population in a health crisis. Veterans have repeatedly celebrated psilocybin's ability to create a sustained change in their mental health and outlook on life. In addition to studies using psilocybin, MAPS has performed extensive MDMA sessions with veterans. As with any psychedelic treatment, however, integrative therapy and post-integration sessions are most beneficial to fully process the experience.

Veteran and psilocybin advocate Chad Kuske suffered for years before finding psilocybin therapy. "I came out of [the psilocybin session] feeling rejuvenated, feeling this massive weight had been lifted off of me that I've been carrying around needlessly for decades," Kuske told *Insider*. "I came out of the session with the desire and the willingness to make the changes necessary to start moving in the other direction. . . . I think the single biggest lasting effect that I've taken away is just a much greater awareness. So, now, instead of reacting to things in life, I can respond. When depression is setting in, or when something angers me or any of the things I used to get frustrated or upset about, I can see it happening."[6]

Many studies show that experiencing a psilocybin session with others who share relatable trauma, as many veterans do, can be an effective treatment for PTSD, making group therapy sessions especially helpful for veterans. To read personal stories from veterans who have suffered severe PTSD and found healing from psilocybin, see the Veteran Voices on the Heroic Hearts Project website.

Overcoming Addiction

With limited resources and effective treatments to overcome it, addiction plays a profound role in today's society. Addictive behaviors are both physical and mental—and, one could argue, emotional as well. Psilocybin has shown promise in this area, particularly with cigarette and alcohol abuse and related disorders such as anorexia nervosa.

One study at John Hopkins tested the effect of one psilocybin dose on cigarette smoking and found an 80 percent abstinence rate after six months and a 60 percent rate at thirty months. As a side note, 86.7 percent of the study subjects rated their psilocybin treatment "among the five most personally meaningful and spiritually significant experiences of their lives."[7]

The Centers for Disease Control and Prevention reports that excessive alcohol consumption kills roughly 95,000 Americans every year, often due to binge drinking or liver disease. In 2022, clinical researcher Michael Bogenshutz conducted a trial to determine psilocybin's effectiveness in combination with protocol psychotherapy for the treatment of alcoholism.[8] The results showed that the combination produced a decrease in the percentage of heavy drinking days in the following thirty-two weeks. The psilocybin group reported 9.7 percent of the days in those thirty-two weeks as heavy drinking days, compared to 26.3 percent in the placebo and psychotherapy group.

As noted by Dr. Walter H. Kaye of the University of California San Diego Eating Disorders Center, "Anorexia nervosa is one of the most difficult to treat conditions we face in psychiatry, with the highest suicide rate of any mental health challenge. . . . Research and progress are urgently needed." In reference to a Johns Hopkins study initiated in 2019, Kaye continued, "We've already seen encouraging data from an exploratory, open-label study in treating anorexia nervosa with COMP360 psilocybin therapy, and this phase II study represents another important step forward."

Bill Wilson, who cofounded Alcoholics Anonymous in 1935, had his first hallucinogenic experience with the prescribed combo of belladonna (*Atropa belladonna*) and henbane (*Hyoscyamus niger*) while in a treatment hospital for severe alcohol abuse. He described the experience as being seized with an ecstasy beyond description and found it profound in his treatment. In 1956 he had his first LSD experience; Wilson was later quoted as saying, "My original spontaneous spiritual experience . . . was enacted with wonderful splendor and conviction," and he thought he "might have found something that could make a big difference to the lives of many who suffered." Currently there are multiple trials running, with positive outcomes published from older studies showing the benefits of psychedelic use in alleviating alcohol addiction.

The Case of Mark

Mark was a white male in his twenties who was living with his parents and working full-time when he enrolled in a clinical psilocybin trial.[9] His binge drinking had begun in his teens and had intensified into adulthood. He reported frequent blackouts and occasional absences from work due to drinking episodes that lasted for days at a time. At baseline, he reported drinking on six of the past eighty-four days, with an average of twenty-two drinks per drinking day. Mark had made multiple unsuccessful attempts at treatment and had attended hundreds of Alcoholics Anonymous meetings. He started the study with the intention of attaining complete abstinence from alcohol, saying, "I just want to stop and have a normal life."

During the first session, Mark encountered his anxiety and fears associated with failure. Though the effects were mild and difficult for him to communicate in words, he said, "It was almost like finding the Holy Grail and the answer to all of life's questions." Self-report assessments revealed that he had experienced a session of moderately high intensity. In the month that followed, Mark remained abstinent and was surprised at how easy this was and how little he thought about alcohol.

Mark's second medication session was higher in both dose and intensity. He was confronted by the harmful effects that his drinking had had on himself and others. He stated, "At one point, I felt I could have cried for joy," when realizing that he was being given "a new slate." In the following weeks, he reported increased motivation and drive, as well as a strong desire to contribute to the world in a meaningful way. He said, "I feel like I'm maturing. Maybe a part of me died when I gave up alcohol."

Mark remained abstinent during the seven months following the second medication session. He opted to have a third open-label medication session with the hope that it would help with his work-related anxiety. He described the experience as "a crash course" in dealing with feelings of disappointment, regret, shame, and unworthiness. He also reported "a couple of eureka moments" and said that the session ended with "calmness, comfort, and reassurance." He said, "I wouldn't be surprised if I never drank again" and added, "I got exactly what I needed out of the experience." One month after this session, he had remained abstinent and expressed a great deal of gratitude for being able to participate in the study. Two years from his initial intake, Mark contacted the study team to report that he had continued to remain abstinent.

Spiritual Growth

As Alan Watts puts it, "Mystical experiences are those peculiar states of consciousness in which the individual discovers himself to be one continuous process with God, with the Universe, with the Ground of Being, or whatever name he may use by cultural conditioning or personal preference for the ultimate and eternal reality."[10] This, in my opinion, has historically been one of the strongest pulls to try psychedelics, whether you seek a deeper connection with your religious faith or deeper meaning.

Walter Pahnke, the clinician in charge of the Good Friday experiment, which we'll discuss in detail in the next chapter, proposed that psilocybin could at times create similar (if not identical) mystical experiences to those recorded in the historical literature of mysticism. In this regard, he viewed the mystical experience as a meta-conscious copresence of God, or any revelatory entity, that promotes the sense of direct connection to God and a deep understanding of that connection.

Psilocybin to Save the Planet

Anyone who knows me well knows that I am happiest in nature. Put me in the woods, on a mountain, at the beach, or outside on my back porch and my inner vibration will rise to its truest self. I feel deeply connected to plants and animals and advocate wildly to protect them, and I am a self-declared biophile.

While I've never met Simon G. Powell, author of *Magic Mushroom Explorer* and many other titles, his work is inspiring and gives a refreshing look into why we might consider using psilocybin. Powell believes that psilocybin gives us a new way to understand life, evolution, and consciousness—it connects us to nature and the environment. There are often moments—if not long stretches of time—when participants in a psilocybin session feel or see the way they are connected to the greater world around them. Having a moment of such deep connection to the Earth can result in radical shifts in one's day-to-day behavior. Simon refers to this connection as the "natural intelligence paradigm."

This place of curiosity during a psilocybin session can help move us from a place where we lack biospherical awareness into a place where our eyes are wide open. When we *feel* connected to something, whether that be a person, animal, or something else in nature, we are more likely to form a positive reciprocal relationship. Scientists have proven that feeling connected makes us feel good. Brain neurotransmitters like endorphins and dopamine release when you feel good, reinforcing that feeling of connectedness. Having a psilocybin experience that promotes a connection to nature and the environment leads to a higher probability that the participant will make changes to maintain a positive relationship with nature. According to Powell, "Psilocybin is an invaluable natural resource for spiritually reviving the human psyche and reconnecting us to the biosphere and the vast intelligence of Nature." Read that again. In the words of Paul Stamets, "If we are able to live in harmony with nature, then we are able to harness nature for these paradigm shifting solutions" (such as addressing climate change).

Why LSD Has Left the Spotlight

....

There are several reasons why psilocybin has supplanted LSD in theraputic applications. From a clinical viewpoint, the duration of LSD's effect results in a much longer session compared to a psilocybin session. There is also a much quicker return to a normal state of mind, which can make the comedown challenging. And, quite honestly, psilocybin doesn't have the historical charge that LSD has. This—combined with the simple fact that psilocybin is difficult to spell, an amusing truth shared with me by Bill Richards—makes psilocybin a softer target in both the political and research worlds.

In *The Sunshine Makers*, a documentary about LSD and psychedelics, we meet two of the biggest producers of LSD and DMT of the 1960s, Nicholas Sand and Tim Scully. While this documentary takes us on a wonderful ride through the psychedelic truth of the era, it is Sand's message that parallels that of Powell: "When you turn on from having a psychedelic session, you tune in to the world around you."

As we move forward on Earth, many believe psychedelics can help us tune in to the environment and promote positive and sustainable change. This deeper connection, as well as the potential to manifest Earth-saving solutions, is another excellent reason to consider psilocybin.

Increasing Creativity and Problem-Solving Ability

Through scientific study, we are witnessing some fascinating ways in which psilocybin turns on our mental, emotional, logical, and creative centers. Enhancing motivation, creativity, and problem-solving in one's professional and personal life have become popular reasons to use psilocybin.

James Fadiman, an incredible leader in this field, has researched the power of psilocybin in creative and artistic endeavors, focusing on methods of using psychedelics that open minds to useful solutions. There is still much we don't know, but Fadiman's research suggests that psilocybin dissolves the obstacles that are often the barriers to finding a solution to a problem. He also notes that psychedelics can give us increased access to unconscious data, more freedom to play spontaneously with hypotheses and paradoxes, and a heightened ability for visualization and fantasy in conjunction with relaxation and decreased anxiety. Basically, psychedelics open the potential to see geometry in space. Combine all of this with the ability to see through false solutions and we increase the chances of finding new solutions to old problems.

A study led by Luisa Procházková from Leiden University in the Netherlands examined whether psilocybin affected participants' ability to think outside the box.[11] Participants were given a set of three tasks, both before and after the ingestion of a microdose of psilocybin. During the study she measured convergent thinking, the identification of a single solution to a problem; fluid intelligence, the capacity to reason and solve new problems; and divergent thinking, the ability to recognize many possible solutions. She also measured the participants' IQ and general analytical abilities before and after ingesting the microdose. Neither IQ nor general analytical ability changed during or after the psilocybin session, but convergent thinking, fluid intelligence, and divergent thinking all increased after psilocybin ingestion. These findings suggest that psilocybin is rather selective in the brain, with one of the greatest effects being on the creative centers.

Engineers, scientists, and members of the tech industry have all been known to utilize psychedelics to increase creativity and look at particularly challenging problems in a new way. It's well known that Steve Jobs used psychedelics, and some say we have the iPhone as a result. His famously said, "Taking LSD was a profound experience, one of the most important things in my life. LSD shows you that there's another side to the coin, and you can't remember it when it wears off, but you know it. It reinforced my sense of what was important—creating great things instead of making money, putting things back into the stream of history and of human consciousness as much as I could."

And consider Kary Mullis, the Nobel Prize winner who developed the polymerase chain reaction, in which a small amount of DNA can be quickly copied to produce large quantities. Once hailed as the greatest discovery of the twentieth century, this technique has allowed scientists to sequence the genomes of humans and thousands of other organisms, leading to important discoveries in medicine and revolutionizing forensics. Mullis was both a unique thinker and a scientist who took psychedelics. He once pondered, "What if I had not taken LSD ever. Would I have still invented PCR? I don't know. I doubt it. I seriously doubt it."[12]

We also see the results of using psychedelics in music and visual art. Alex and Allyson Grey, who met on an acid trip in 1976, have spearheaded the Visionary Art movement, which is based on the premise that art is a manifestation of the divine within. Psychidelic use "encourages the development of our inner sight," Alex Grey has said. "To find the visionary realm, we use the intuitive inner eye: The eye of contemplation; the eye of the soul. All the inspiring ideas we have as artists originate here."

Barriers to Use

I feel it is important to note that barriers exist for a large number of people here in the United States to have access to psilocybin and a safe space in which to use it. Psilocybin is making its way into mainstream news, and multiple states are working to decriminalize its use. An abundance of research has shown psilocybin can be used to successfully treat PTSD and other mental health issues. However, many of us over the age of forty have lived through a lot of propaganda and stigmatized messaging regarding psilocybin. Such messaging is still trickling down and

WHY PEOPLE USE PSILOCYBIN ✦ 51

impacting younger generations as well. It can be confusing and challenging when outdated messaging gets in the way of potential healing, and this stigma can require a great deal of deprogramming before even considering experiencing a psilocybin session.

When we educate ourselves on the history of psychedelics, which I will dive into in Chapter 3, another area may make some readers uncomfortable. White readers of this book must come to terms with the institutionalized and structural biases cemented into the history of psychedelics. Although we may not have individually acted to perpetrate racist acts within the psychedelic space, by not actively naming and changing the narrative, we have become complicit in these problems. While many tout the "all-encompassing love and acceptance" of psychedelics, it has quickly become apparent that racial biases are still present. I urge you to give this paragraph some thought and consider how your own personal biases, conscious and subconscious, affect the space moving forward.

We also have states, like Oregon, where people are launching into psilocybin capitalistic endeavors. Some companies have identified the potential windfall this new opportunity could provide but lack the necessary education or ethics to properly deliver psilocybin therapy. This can easily trigger preconceived notions about whether psilocybin is safe or not. Some see the road paved as an open door to cultural acceptance, whereas others see the rise of entrepreneurial psilocybin endeavors as a reason to avoid it. With the media playing a major role in psilocybin's return to society, it can be very challenging to decipher what we, as individuals, truly believe about how and why to use it. This entrepreneurial approach also creates financial barriers to use. Do a quick Google search and you'll quickly see the *average* cost of a psilocybin session or retreat runs $3000 to $10,000 or more. I don't think I need to point out the barrier here. Deconstructing old messaging, stereotyping, and barriers to accessibility will be necessary to ensure the success of psilocybin therapy.

Summary

While the above list of reasons to try psychedelics is by no means exhaustive, maybe it helps to aim your compass. While research has shown psilocybin therapy to be of benefit to those suffering from trauma, PTSD, anxiety, and addiction, that is just the tip of the iceberg of its usefulness. If your reason for wanting to have a psilocybin session is not mentioned here, trust that it is just as valid as the rest. Shedding the old thought patterns of what psychedelics are, how they affect us, and imprinted societal stereotyping will be crucial as we move toward the broader acceptance of this healing medicine. Over 21 million Americans over the age of eighteen are experiencing mental health difficulties, and what we are doing isn't working. There is a need for change. When we distill the reasons why we are drawn to psilocybin therapy, we find the desire for knowledge and connection. This may feel like different things to different people—connection to oneself, to others, to healing, to your purpose, to your work, to potential beyonds, or to the Earth. As an inscription at St. Paul's Monastery on Mt. Athos in Greece says, "If you die before you die, then you won't die when you die."

CHAPTER 3

History of Psilocybin

FROM THE FAR CORNERS OF THE WORLD—Africa to Mesoamerica to Europe—there is a rich history of psilocybin use. As we move into that discussion, let us start by honoring the past. I want to first acknowledge the mushrooms for the healing potential they offer us. Centuries of psilocybin use has led to healing, divine manifestation, and vision.

Next I want to acknowledge all the lineage holders of this traditionally sacred fungi. Without them we'd likely have no connection to this medicine. Because of this, I say thank you, thank you, thank you. These lineage holders sacrificed so much to honor and preserve the traditions, beliefs, customs, and rituals they knew to be true, despite the fact that the caring and holding of this medicine often led to violence. Understanding how colonization has affected ceremonial and indigenous uses of psychedelics is important as we move into the future of psychedelic space.

I say thank you to all of those who came before me and carried the burdens of this healing medicine so that you and I can have access to it.

Psilocybin Around the World

Looking through the lens of Western psilocybin history, we are often first pointed to the stories of R. Gordon Wasson, María Sabina, and ethnobotanist Richard Schultes. But the full picture is much broader, encompassing Mesoamerican, Mexican, and African traditions, the Eleusian ceremonies of ancient Greece, and the history of witchcraft in Europe and the British Isles just as a start.

Shamans

....

Shamanism is a system of religious practice historically associated with indigenous and tribal society. Many cultures believe in a multidimensional existence, and it is the shaman's role to travel into these places and spaces to receive messages and help as needed, acting as the primary mediator between humans and these other worlds. A medicine woman/man can also be a shaman, but some traditions separate the two. A medicine person's role is as the primary healer of physical disease through cultural tools and traditional techniques. Both roles were historically passed down by lineage, apprenticeship, spirit quest, or miraculous experience.

The word *shaman* comes from Evenki, a Tungusic language: *sˇaman* or *xaman*, meaning "agitated," "excited," or "raised." In Siberia, where the term originated, music and sound are often integral aspects of shamanism. The use of drums and other instruments, including singing, are the means to connect to the other worlds and spirits.

Why have I included psilocybin history in this book? Well, because it is important. Much of today's psychedelic training curricula are still educating facilitators about psilocybin in a colonized way. Breaking down this old way of thinking is imperative, now more than ever, as the modern psychedelic model emerges. The true history of psilocybin use is conveyed through the oral tradition of lineage holders, ancient written documentation, and ethnomycological evidence from various experts, but determining with certainty who was the original sacred holder of the medicinal fungi is a difficult question to answer. Hopefully the information in this chapter provides enough context for you to appreciate how long psilocybin has been used for healing, guidance, spiritualism, protection, and inner knowledge.

The shaman, as a spiritual practitioner, uses drums, rattles, hallucinogens, or other devices in the course of a ritual session, entering an altered state (sometimes also called a trance) in order to establish contact with spiritual forces in the other world. The goal of this spiritual encounter is to secure the help of spiritual beings that populate this otherworldly reality to resolve a problem, cure a patient, correct a misfortune, or predict the future.

Since the word *shaman* was introduced into Western usage in the eighteenth century, it has meant various things to different people. Mircea Eliade, a historian of religion and author of *Shamanism: Archaic Techniques of Ecstasy*, viewed shamanism as the earliest form of religion. Unfortunately, Eliade generalized the term *shaman* to refer to all healers across the globe that conduct or offer ceremonies to heal. Although many scholars now believe that ecstasy (an altered state) is not a necessary attribute of shamanism, for many Western seekers it is one of the basic pillars of this spiritual practice.

Mushrooms, including bioactive species, have been a resource to humans since the Pliocene.[1] Due to mushrooms' ability to spread their spores far and wide, it is quite possible that *Psilocybe* (as well as other psychedelic fungi) existed across the world—particularly if you consider the Pangaea theory that all the planet's landmasses were once connected. We can imagine that these psychedelic fungi were ingested by foraging societies around the world simultaneously upon discovery.

Researchers José Manuel Rodríguez Arce and Michael Winkelman have suggested that psilocybin played a role in human evolution.[2] While some ancient foragers may have discovered psilocybin and disregarded it, others found and ingested it, experiencing the medicine's great mystery, connection, and self-exploration. It is these peoples who created unique relationships and ceremonies with the magic mushroom that still persist in many cultures today.

Mexico and Central America

When researching various histories of psilocybin use, I discovered the wonderful book *Women and Knowledge in Mesoamerica: From East L.A. to Anahuac* by Paloma Martinez-Cruz. My Western psychedelic education offered very little in the way of cultural history of psilocybin, and I did not want to regurgitate the Western stories of psychedelic discovery through cultural appropriation. The Mesoamerican history holds some of the strongest records of psilocybin use, and Martinez-Cruz's book offers incredible insight into the ways in which women were the holders of the knowledge and wisdom.

When reading her work, I was particularly struck by the limitations of my own conditioning. As Martinez-Cruz so eloquently put it, if we only consider ideas and concepts based on the empirical-critical model, we have already been derailed. Colonialist ideals have often recast concepts, traditions, and beliefs to "fit" into a limited understanding, but the Mesoamerican history should not be told from a perspective in which it did not operate.

The history of psilocybin use in Mesoamerica begins more than 3500 years ago, during the Olmec times. The Olmecs' way of living wove together an intricate relationship between the human body, nature, and cosmology. The Mesoamerican relationship with psilocybin is often linked to the Creator/Wind God Quetzalcoatl. In the *Codex Mexicanus I*, an accordion-folded pre-Columbian piece of Mixtec writing, there are representations of Quetzalcoatl in ceremony with Xochipilli and Tezcatlipoca and mushroom representations. Gastón Guzmán Huerta, a Mexican mycologist and educator, also identified *Psilocybe zapotecorum* symbolism on clay figurines from the Capacha culture of Colima, where individuals with serpent-like arms stand together venerating the mushroom and a traditional healer, which Guzmán Huerta identified as Quetzalcoatl.[3]

Aztec psilocybin history is centered around Xochipilli, the god of art, games, dance, flowers, and song. Although this deity is often attributed to the Aztec culture, he appears to predate them. In Nahuatl, the language spoken by the Mexica, Xochipilli means "Flower Prince." The Aztecs had a long history of using psychedelics in ceremony and ritual, particularly teotlnanácatl, the "sacred mushroom" or "god's flesh mushroom" (scholars still debate whether teotlnanácatl was *Psilocybe aztecorum* or *Psilocybe mexicana*). A statue from the late postclassical period (1450 to 1500 CE) shows Xochipilli adorned with what is presumed to be psychotropic flowers, animal skins, and teotlnanácatl.

In his sixteenth-century book *Historia de las cosas de Nueva España*, Jesuit missionary Bernardino de Sahagún provided written documentation of magic mushrooms: "There are some small mushrooms in that region which are called teonanácatl; these grow under the grass (hay) of the fields and pastures. They are round, having a rather high stipe, slender and terete. When eaten, they have a bad taste, hurting the throat, and they cause intoxication. They are medicinal for fevers and for rheumatism. Only two or three need to be eaten. Those who eat them see visions and feel a faintness of the heart. And they provoke to lust those who eat a number, or even a few, of them."

In 1656, Francisco Hernández de Toledo, a physician to the king of Spain, recorded the use of psilocybin by the Aztecs, both in and outside of ceremonial use. As someone who did not partake in or understand the psilocybin experience, he recorded participants reacting as if temporarily mad with hallucinations and visions. The Aztecs' rituals, which were integral to their way of life, were rejected and considered tribal by the Spaniards, to be punished by death should they continue. As a result, psilocybin's use had to be hidden away.

Psilocybin is also a part of the Mayan culture, whose advances in architecture, astronomy, medicine, and math are renowned—and perhaps inspired by the ceremonial uses of psychedelics. This Mesoamerican civilization occupied a nearly continuous territory spanning southern Mexico, Guatemala, and northern Belize. Stone mushroom statues have been found in Guatemala, and representations of mushroom use in Mayan religious ceremonies have been recorded. In *Hallucinogens and Culture*, Peter T. Furst noted that "as long as 3000 years ago at least the inhabitants of the highlands and the Pacific slope of Guatemala, as well as some of their neighbors, held certain mushrooms to be so sacred and powerful—perhaps even divine—that they represented them in great numbers in sculptured stone."

The Mazatec people are an indigenous group from the mountains of Oaxaca, Mexico. Their origin is difficult to trace, but they seem to have occupied the Sierra Madre Occidental in central Mexico from as early as the twelfth century. Through cultural beliefs and shamanism, the Mazatec use ritual and ceremony to commune with spirits, divine information, heal ailments, and open the lines of communication with the divine. These rituals are popularly known as veladas and the community healers, who use powerful visionary plants like *Psilocybe* mushrooms and *Salvia divinorum*, are curanderas. The Mazatec believe that the mushrooms' energies contain helpful spirits for the person/community they are being called for and that the mushrooms are so pure of spirit that only children can harvest them. The mushrooms are viewed as sacred beings that have come to help, and the Mazatec work to establish a reciprocal relationship of gratitude and respect with them. In Oaxaca, the majority of healers who have reached the highest stature of wisdom and truth are women. To better understand historical use of psilocybin in Mexican cultures, I encourage you to seek out the works of Gastón Guzmán Huerta, who researched, wrote, and educated on the subject of mycology for a large part of his life.

Of the curanderas, Paloma Martinez-Cruz wonders, "Is the Mazatec mushroom ritual, and the healer women that officiate this ritual, an indigenous resistance to colonial oppression?"

Dr. Salvador Roquet is an important figure in modern psychedlic therapy. A psychiatrist, Roquet began administering psychedelic substances to his patients in 1967. While there are questions regarding his techniques—portions of his therapy sessions involved extreme amounts of stimulation—Roquet's work contributed to many of the theories and practices of Western psychedelic research models. Stan Grof and Bill Richards, significant contributors to the field of psychedelic medicine, met with Roquet in 1972 and participated in a session with him.

Africa

The 1995 discovery of *Psilocybe natalensis* in the Natal region of South Africa verified that psychedelic mushrooms are indigenous to Africa. Mycologist Darren Springer (www.darrenlebaron.com), provides a compendious look at how psilocybin mushrooms first originated on the African continent in many of his lectures and classes. His interest in the subject began when he first saw a world map marked with tiny dots showing where all the psychedelic mushrooms could be found in the world. Smack dab in the middle was the huge landmass of Africa. Other regions had numerous dots over them, but Africa only had six—just six tiny little dots over this entire large continent.

According to Springer, the initial explanation for the apparently low occurrence of African psychoactives was easy to identify. Historically, mycological research in Africa has not been popular, research funding has not been readily available, and the preconceived notion that Africa can be difficult to navigate made it a less-than-favorable choice for scientists. Despite this, some mycologists and ethnobotanists have succeeded in conducting research across the continent and have reported some wonderful discoveries.

Believe it or not, 9000 to 7000 years ago the area of the Sahara Desert was a bountiful environment that easily supported human life. When I traveled there in 2007 it was quite easy to picture such an existence, particularly walking the white desert and witnessing the rocks carved by wind and water. We know through radiocarbon dating that the cave art found in this area matches up with this time period. The images depict flowers, gardens, food, animals, and people. In the lower caves you can see images of everyday life, but as you move up to higher altitude caves there are images that represent gods, spirits, and mythical beings.

Comparisons have been made between the Saharan images and those found in Mexico: both show people, some wearing horns or horn-type headdresses, dancing next to mushrooms and people with mushroom heads. In the Paleolithic murals of the cave walls of Tin-Tazarift at Tassili N'Ajjer in Algeria images of masked anthropomorphic beings engage in ecstatic dancing. Another image shows humanoid figures that are dancing or running and carrying mushrooms, which are connected by dotted lines to their heads, perhaps indicating the influence of the mushrooms on their minds. These murals are some of the most famous archeological evidence of the presence of psychedelic mushrooms in Africa.

Many believe that the psychedelic mushrooms containing psilocybin were a part of Egyptian culture and ceremonial tradition. In the Egyptian *Book of the Dead*, mushrooms are called "the food of the gods," "celestial food," and "flesh of the gods." The mushrooms were typically only ingested by the upper class and during ceremonial or religious events. There are countless images of mushrooms in the temples throughout Egypt, and they are often depicted in baskets or pouches or being shared among people. Archaeologists have also found ceremonial pouches filled with mushrooms that were buried with the dead to assist them in their journey to the afterlife. Osiris, the Egyptian god of the underworld, is also believed to be the personification of the psilocybin mushroom. Gods, goddesses, and rulers and for religious ceremonies were depicted wearing single, double, and triple crowns in specific colors, and ethnobotanist Stephen Berlant claims white triple crowns represented the psilocybin mushroom.[4]

Researchers including Gastón Guzmán Huerta, Stuart C. Nixon, Florencia Ramírez Guillén, Alonso Cortés-Pérez, and Giorgio Samorini have all dedicated time and contemplative energy to studying the use of psilocybin in Africa. Darren Springer also offers a class focused on the topic.

Greece

The Eleusinian Mysteries were a set of secret religious rites—the Lesser and Greater Mysteries—that took place annually in Greece from 1450 BCE to 392 CE. Many believe it was the consumption of psychedelics in a communal drink, known as the *kykeon*, that led initiates to spiritual transformation and illumination. In *The Road to Eleusis: Unveiling the Secret of the Mysteries*, R. Gordon Wasson, Albert Hofmann, and Carl A. P. Ruck go in depth as to why they believe it was a psychedelic substance used in the ceremonial drink.

The Greater Mysteries ceremony was centered around Demeter, the goddess of agriculture and the fertility of the earth, and her daughter Persephone and was held around the autumnal equinox each year. The rites were based at the Sanctuary of Eleusis, and it was said that "the life of the Greeks [would be] unlivable, if they were prevented from properly observing the most sacred Mysteries, which hold the whole human race together."[5] The initiates would gather for the ritual at a specific starting point and begin their walk on the "road to Eleusis." The *kykeon* would be consumed, and by the time they entered the ritual site, "something" would be revealed. That something has led to a lot of debate. A vision of Demeter perhaps? Enlightenment? A connection to a greater power? Unfortunately, we will never know.

Britain and Ireland

Some of my favorite reflections on psilocybin use have to do with its history in the British Isles. For instance, Kathryn Solie has written extensively on psychedelics and witch history. As someone who feels akin to rituals, herbal medicine, and tradition, I've always held a fascination with the history of Druids and priestess culture, which can also include the history of witchcraft. Specialized knowledge in healing and plant medicine was at the core of these communities, and it's not surprising that psilocybin was one of the many tools they used in their healing practices. It is commonly thought that the flying ointments of the past included psilocybin; by spreading this ointment over their bodies, the women who made it would soon be "flying" into the sky.

The Druids have a long history of using psychedelics, and both liberty cap (*Psilocybe semilanceata*) and fly agaric mushrooms (*Amanita muscaria*) grow in Ireland. The Druids believe that consuming these mushrooms brings great knowledge and insight, as they are a direct way to communicate with the gods. Historically, they understood that mushrooms were just the small fruit of a gigantic underground fungi. By consuming them they are able to receive messages from the Earth and tap into the world in a unique way. The art in the caves of Knowth and Newgrange depict a spiral motif that some have theorized is a representation of the psychedelic state.

In Andy Letcher's book *Shroom: A Cultural History of the Magic Mushroom*, he shares a handful of nineteenth-century medical accounts of accidental psilocybin intoxication. These London residents suddenly found themselves in a psychedelic state after eating what they thought were normal culinary fungi. Many of these accounts will provide a little chuckle, as the unknowing patients succumbed to fits of giddiness and reported seeing the wallpaper come alive. Despite zero deaths reported from the ingestion of psychedelic mushrooms, they were lumped into the purely toxic mushroom group. Such occurrences began to weave an underlying thread that all mushrooms could make you crazy, poison you, or bring you to your death, leading to the general notion that mushrooms were to be avoided.

An interesting endnote to this part of history was that as a result of these accidental "poisonings," members of London's mycology clubs decided to devise a proper identification system for mushrooms. Their new system classified mushrooms based on both spore color and gill type, which elevated mushrooms' identification status to that of the plant kingdom. The original system included psychedelic mushrooms, but these types began to disappear from field guides in the early twentieth century. Some proposed that the "toxic" label made these mushrooms seem unfit for use, and over time, they were omitted as worthless.

Archeological Evidence of Psychedelic Mushroom Use

....

Our search for altered states of consciousness has had a long history.

The earliest evidence of psychedelic mushroom use is a mural found in northern Australia that depicts people with mushroom heads and what is believed to be an illustration of a psychedelic trance. Archeologists have dated it back to 10,000 BCE.

The Selva Pascuala cave mural in Spain, dating to 4000 BCE, is the oldest known illustration of psilocybin mushrooms in Europe. Based on the bull in the mural, archeologists believe the mushrooms are *Psilocybe hispanica*, which grows in the region and often emerges from animal dung.

Ötzi (a.k.a. the Iceman), the mummy of a man who lived between 3400 and 3100 BCE near the present-day border of Austria and Italy, was found with two types of mushrooms.

According to the pre-Columbian *Codex Vindobonensis*, mind-altering mushrooms were used in religious ceremonies in ancient Mexico. Roman Catholic priests also observed and recorded the consumption of hallucinogenic mushrooms by native peoples after the conquest of Mexico in 1519.

American History of Psilocybin

Cave and stone art, artifacts, and preserved specimens provide archeological evidence that psilocybin has been used for millennia in North and South America. In European culture, however, the fear that mushrooms could either make you crazy or kill you led early American settlers to be hesitant to adopt the Mesoamerican and American Indian ceremonial use of psychedelics. This fear, disregard, and refusal to learn from Indigenous cultures created prejudices and a foundation for racial injustices that have lasted for centuries.

The modern-day American relationship with psilocybin is centered around R. Gordon Wasson's work. Almost every book you read will mention Wasson and his wife Valentina, as well as their quest to understand cultural variances regarding mushrooms. But his work and relationship with María Sabina is where Western history begins. Sabina was a Mazatec curandera who, as a young child in Oaxaca, was called to be a guide, healer, ceremonialist, and holder of this sacred medicine.[6] Wasson was an American banker and amateur mycologist with a passion for natural history. In 1957, he published an article titled "Seeking the Magic Mushroom" in *Life* magazine, in which he described his participation in a Mazatec psilocybin ritual with Sabina two years earlier. Wasson and his colleague, New York society photographer Allan Richardson, were some of the first Westerners to participate in the ceremony.

Wasson's article set off a cascade of immense interest in psychedelic mushrooms in the United States. Not only did massive numbers of people begin to travel to Oaxaca in search of the mushrooms, but research ramped up quickly. All of this exploitation was done with little to no consideration of the impacts it would have on Sabina, her town, their medicine, or their traditions. While Wasson had commented that psilocybin must be treated with great reverence and was not to be eaten for excitement or recreation, he failed to protect Sabina's anonymity. Instead, he took the knowledge she graciously offered and disseminated it widely. The traditions, ceremony, and reverence of the Mazatec culture was quickly forgotten. All that Americans heard was that there was a mushroom in Mexico that one could eat to reach enlightenment. Years later, Wasson expressed regret over the publicity the essay brought to the Mazatec as well as the desecration of the mushroom ritual. While his intentions may have been innocent, Wasson's actions brought a flood of intruders and a claim of ownership to something not rightfully his to offer.

When Wasson returned home from Oaxaca, he sent some of the mushrooms to Dr. Andrija Puharich, who analyzed them and identified the chemicals responsible for their hallucinogenic effects; Wasson also ingested some and shared them with others. Roger Heim, a French botanist, took great interest in Wasson's work and they began traveling together to Mexico. It was Heim who collected samples of Mexican Psilocybe mushrooms and gave them to Albert Hofmann, the chemist who had discovered LSD. At the time, Hofmann was working for the pharmaceutical company Sandoz. With his background and passion for psychedelic medicine, he worked diligently until he isolated and identified psilocybin and psilocin as the active principal alkaloids of *Psilocybe*. Hofmann synthesized psilocybin in the form of 4-AcO-DET in 1958. Sandoz patented the drug and the extraction process, labeled it Indocybin, and marketed it to doctors around the world. The fact that the Mazatec people were offered no rights to or monetary compensation for what was once theirs must be acknowledged. As we move through the history of psilocybin, we need to always consider the ways in which this medicine did not originate in the Western world nor should we stake claim to it.

On the flipside, the infamous *Life* magazine article set the wheels set in motion for American psilocybin interest, inspiring the likes of Timothy Leary, Terence McKenna, Richard Alpert, and Ralph Metzner, to name a few, to carve out a new path in their professional careers and ultimately creating one of the biggest shifts in modern psychedelic history. Research in psychedelic medicine surged as a result, but it was the effect on the general public that was most astounding. What was this crazy mushroom that allowed you to see God, to see yourself, to feel connected like you never had before? To teach you not to be afraid of death, how to love yourself and love others openly? The United States was at the precipice of a tumultuous period marked by the Civil Rights Movement and the Vietnam War. People—especially young people—were begging for a new way to understand the world, and Wasson's article proved there was one.

Massive numbers of people went to Mexico to seek the message they had heard about, signaling the dawn of psychedelic tourism. These Americans wanted enlightenment, understanding, connection, and peace. This new awareness also led to the dawning of mushroom seeking in the United States. As it turned out, *Psilocybe* species also grew. Once wild-crafting native species closer to home took hold, people began experimenting with home cultivation.

Those who encouraged the use of psychedelics at that time believed that ingesting them led to new perspectives in spiritual growth, self-love, and connection to others. We can refer to them as the Western pioneers of psychedelic medicine. Osmond, McKenna, Leary, Alpert, Metzner, and many others were encouraging the population to explore the horizons of what psychedelics could offer. The early leaders in the Western psychedelic movement were doing something that hadn't been done before. They were raising awareness of the benefits of psychedelics within an academic context. Timothy Leary, the Harvard professor once labeled as the "most dangerous man in America," believed young adults should explore their spirituality with the use of psychedelics outside of traditional religious norms.

Richard Alpert (now known as Ram Dass), another Harvard professor, teamed up with Leary to conduct research with both LSD and psilocybin to explore spirituality and mystical experiences. These studies created a platform which would be expanded on for years to come. Despite criticism that exploring psilocybin without proper supervision was potentially dangerous, their work revolutionized youth to "turn on, turn in, drop out."

As a result, the country witnessed a change in the collective perception and the rise of the psychedelic 1960s. Many of these pioneers had ways to reach large groups of young people, and they viewed their experiences on psilocybin and LSD as life-changing and life-affirming. Allen Ginsberg's psilocybin use fueled much of his antiwar and nonviolent rebellion. *The Electric Kool-Aid Acid Test*, Tom Wolfe's account of the journey of Ken Kesey, the Merry Pranksters, and a jar of LSD-laced orange juice is said to be the mythological starting point of Western psychedelic history. Musical artists such as Bob Dylan, the Beatles, and the Grateful Dead all openly spoke of their use of psychedelics and the influence it had on their music. Their thousands of listeners got the message that psychedelics can set you free.

Clinical research was clicking along. Psilocybin research was alive and well throughout the 1960s and 1970s, as the number of research papers submitted with positive outcomes soared.

On Good Friday in 1962, at Boston University's Marsh Chapel, Walter Pahnke performed a double-blind trial, giving twenty theological students either 30 mg of synthetic psilocybin or 200 mg of niacin as a placebo. At the same time, African American author, minister, and educator Howard Thurman presided over the congregation. As Thurman delivered the Good Friday service, the students listened below in a small worship space. Every student who received psilocybin reported having a mystical experience, whereas those in the control group simply became flushed for a couple hours due to the niacin placebo. The cause of the participants mystical experience has been much debated. Perhaps it was the participants' religious backgrounds, the spiritual environment, or the sermon's reverent message. But in a follow-up study conducted twenty-five years later, a majority of participants still reported the Good Friday experiment as one of the most profound experiences of their life.

Bill Richards was one of my professors and is one of the leading American psychedelic researchers. From 1967 to 1977, he conducted studies at the Maryland Psychiatric Research Center, focusing on the treatment of alcoholism, heroin addiction, depression, and anxiety in terminally ill cancer patients using psychedelics. While his clinical work mostly focused on how to alleviate clinically defined conditions, he had a passion for learning about the mystical experiences psychedelics can elicit. (Check out Richards's book *Sacred Knowledge: Psychedelics and Religious Experiences* to learn more about his clinical path with psychedelics—it's a fun and interesting read.)

Unfortunately, not everyone was open to the idea of pursuing deeper levels of consciousness. The United States is a society dictated by norms, and psychedelics at the time were most definitely outside the norm. The messaging in mass media and religious and political realms was that psychedelics were turning our good kids into crazy, out-of-control heathens. Much of what was disseminated was either completely made up or was misinformation drawn from scientific studies designed to find damaging, harmful effects. Anyone who used psychedelics was ostracized and deemed dangerous, criminal, and unfit for normal society. Yet those who tried psilocybin reported it giving them the courage to have an independent perspective on life. Here was an opportunity to learn more about themselves, each other, and the world. Many people, groups, and politicians were desperate for psychedelics to go away so they could reject this new way of thinking and maintain the status quo.

As psychedelics became more and more politicized, legal action followed—leading to the classification of psilocybin as a Schedule I drug in 1968 and the outlawing of psychedelics in 1970. While the oft-repeated tale of Richard Nixon calling Timothy Leary "the most dangerous man in America" happens not to be true, it has persisted as myth because it feels true to the atmosphere of the time. Despite all types of Americans experiencing psychedelics and despite them doing their best to share the positive outcomes, it fell on deaf ears.

By the late 1970s, federal funding for psychedelic research had dwindled and American academic institutions began discouraging research and limiting access for those who were interested. At the Maryland Psychiatric Research Center, Richards was the last man standing. In 1977, as he administered a dose of psilocybin to one of his participants, he thought his career in psychedelic research was over. Disheartened not just for his career, but for the countless number of people he knew psilocybin could help, he pondered what may come next for him. After years of successful clinical trials and witnessing life-changing results, psilocybin research, he feared, had taken its last breath.

But Richards never gave up hope, and neither did a strong contingency of professionals who have continued to advocate for the right to administer psychedelic medicine. After more than two dormant decades, in 1999, Richards and his colleague Roland R. Griffiths finally received FDA approval to conduct new psilocybin research. This rebirth started at Johns Hopkins University, with studies focused on relieving terminal diagnosis stress and anxiety centered around the dying experience for cancer patients.

Today, organizations like the Heffter Research Institute promote research with psychedelics, and private funding for clinical trials is now available. Heffter researchers believe that the unexplored potential of psychedelics requires careful scientific research to find their best uses in medical treatment. COMPASS Pathways is a pharmaceutical and biotechnology company leading the way through research with a focus on treatment-resistant depression. Currently many states are considering proposals that would legalize the medical use of psilocybin. In the meantime, you can check out the website clinicaltrials.gov (enter "psilocybin" in the Other Terms field) to see a list of trials that are currently recruiting participants.

Psilocybin Use and Cultural Appropriation

Appropriation is the action of taking something for one's own use, typically without the owner's permission, whereas *cultural appropriation* is the inappropriate or unacknowledged adoption of an element or elements of one culture or identity by members of another culture or identity.

We must acknowledge that most white Americans of European descent have no cultural connection to psilocybin or the ceremonial uses of it. This cultural heritage does not include how, why, or when to use it. As psilocybin moves into legal use across the United States, it is imperative to educate ourselves on its origins and cultural history, as

Important Figures in
Psilocybin History

....

Ram Dass (Richard Alpert; d. 2019) Psychedelic proponent and researcher in the 1960s turned meditation guru

James Fadiman Writer, researcher, and lecturer known for his work on microdosing psychedelics

Stan Grof Psychiatrist with over sixty years of experience in the research of non-ordinary states of consciousness

Albert Hofmann (d. 2008) Swiss chemist known for being the first to synthesize, ingest, and learn the psychedelic effects of LSD; Hofmann's team also isolated, named, and synthesized the principal mushroom psychedelic compounds, psilocybin and psilocin

Gastón Guzmán Huerta (d. 2016) Mexican mycologist and anthropologist who was an authority on the genus *Psilocybe*

Aldous Huxley (d. 1963) Writer, philosopher, and author of *The Doors of Perception*

Timothy Leary (d. 1996) Psychologist and author known for his strong advocacy of psychedelic drugs

Terence McKenna (d. 2000) Ethnobotanist and mystic who advocated for the responsible use of naturally occurring psychedelic plants

Ralph Metzner (d. 2019) Psychologist, writer, and researcher who participated in psychedelic research at Harvard University in the early 1960s with Timothy Leary and Richard Alpert

Walter Pahnke (d. 1971) Minister, physician, and psychiatrist most famous for the Good Friday Experiment conducted at Boston University in 1962

Janis Phelps Founder and director of the CIIS Center for Psyche-delic Therapies and Research program

Simon G. Powell British writer who focuses on the topics of biophilia and psilocybin

Bill Richards Author, researcher, and psychologist at Johns Hopkins University School of Medicine

Carl A. P. Ruck Professor of Classical Studies at Boston University, author of *The Road to Eleusis*

María Sabina (d. 1985) Mazatec curandera, shaman, and poet who lived in Huautla de Jiménez, Oaxaca; known for working with R. Gordon Wasson

Ben Sessa Writer, psychiatrist, and researcher who focuses on addiction, adolescent care, and psychedelics

Alexander "Sasha" and Ann Shulgin (Alexander d. 2014) Alexander was an American medicinal chemist credited with introducing 3,4-methylenedioxymethamphetamine (MDMA) to psychologists in the late 1970s; as a couple, they advocated for the use of halluci-nogens in psychotherapy and documented their experiences with hundreds of drugs in two widely read books, *PiHKAL* and *TiHKAL*

Paul Stamets Mycologist, medical researcher, author, and entre-preneur who is considered an intellectual and industry leader in medicinal fungi

R. Gordon Wasson (d. 1986) American banker and amateur mycolo-gist who participated in a mushroom ritual with María Sabina and subsequently published the article "Seeking the Magic Mushroom" in *Life* magazine

well as acknowledge the historical racism and biases that accompany it. Due to the combined factors of research, veteran support, and the public drive for legalization, we will most likely see the psychedelic landscape change dramatically in our lifetimes. We need to shape the future of this medicine and with these thoughts in mind.

The conversation of ethics and ethical use of psychedelics is where I often experience a moderate swing of thoughts, feelings, justifications, guilt, honor, and straight-up confusion. When I first dove into being a psychedelic facilitator, there were only a couple of things that I felt sure about. First, I wasn't a shaman. I've worked with The Foundation for Shamanic Studies founded by Michael Harner, learned with a shaman in Peru, been inducted in the ways of Mayan spiritual medicine, learned from Alberto Villoldo, and have spent countless years learning various traditions and practices. But I've never felt that made me a shaman. The second thing I knew was that my heart and soul has always felt connected to the wonders of nature. Nature has consistently provided me with sustenance for the body and mind. I have always followed the call when nature speaks, and the lessons I've learned have shaped me as a human. I realize that might sound a bit too far out for some of you, but I have received whispers from the trees about which way to go when I've been lost in the woods and been warned by many animals when danger was ahead. (If you'd like to explore this concept more deeply, read *The Spell of the Sensuous* by David Abram.) I believe we all have the ability to listen to the world around us, but it can be hard to hear sometimes because our world and our own internal thoughts are so loud.

When we reflect on the historical uses and traditions of psilocybin, we must take into account the cultures that have used psilocybin as part of their customs for centuries. (Synthesized medicines like MDMA and LSD are a different story.) To me, there are clear delineations when it comes to sacred medicine. The American Indians' connection to peyote and the South American peoples' relationship with San Pedro and ayahuasca are clear examples of indigenous plants providing for the communities in which they grow. These plants are seen as valuable medicine to be used in traditional ceremonies of their culture. I believe the cultures who hold the lineage have the right to these medicines and that they should be the ones to decide who harvests and uses them. (This is my opinion, and I am fully aware of how charged this topic can be.)

Many cultures have a very different relationship to nature than we do in the United States. After a one-time chance encounter, I was invited to visit Slovenia, a tiny country I'd never heard of. Upon my arrival I was quickly enamored with Slovenian culture, which regards poetry and music as two of the most coveted professions. The people I met in Slovenia valued nature as a religion. In Slavic mythology, god is a mountain referred to as Father Triglav and and its power is deeply rooted in the soil and all that comes from it.

Mazatecs believe the *Psilocybe* mushrooms are like spirit children, pure and unadulterated by negativity. The practice of harvesting them is sacred and a ceremony unto itself. There are intentions, procedures, songs, and so much more that goes into truly connecting and understanding the medicine at the time of harvest and preparation. I completely agree with this mode of thinking and believe in the energetics of plants and medicine. Everything holds an energetic charge—it's basic physics, folks! As always, anything can sway more to the positive or the negative based on the environment it has existed in.

So when we move into discussions regarding who has the right to use these medicines, we need to sit with the thoughts and considerations from a cultural perspective. While María Sabina made the choice to share her sacred medicine, it is hard to hear her story and not feel a disproportionate advantage on the part of R. Gordon Wasson. The subsequent return of Wasson to the United States, where psilocybin samples were turned over to be isolated in a lab, is when I believe we entered into cultural appropriation territory. Did Sabina grant Wasson permission to do this? What if he had instead returned home and sought out a local North American Psyilocybe species? What if he'd offered compensation to Sabina (and her village or community) in the form of rights to the commercially produced drug or regular cash payouts on the profits?

And because *Psilocybe* grows almost worldwide (fly little spores, fly!), does any single culture own it? These are the ramblings of a concerned psychedelic facilitator.

So I pose the question: Is using psilocybin cultural appropriation? Some say yes, and others, no. When we look to cultural leaders who have had a longer history with psilocybin, some say take it and use it, as it is for the benefit of all. Others have strongly opposed its use by those who are not lineage holders. After sitting through countless conversations and wrestling with this idea for myself, this is where I have landed personally. Because of my personal journey, I feel called to work and share what I know regarding psilocybin medicine. I've seen too much suffering in my life not to. I've witnessed too much healing from the use of these substances not to. I think of my brother almost every day, wishing he'd had the opportunity to use psychedelics in an attempt to beat the addiction that eventually took his life. Has a tribal leader or person of cultural origin looked me in the eye and granted me a blessing to use psilocybin freely in the world? No, but I have been gifted the mushrooms themselves time and time again and have been asked to help others in need. Because of this, I move forward in an attempt to be of service. But each and every time I use psilocybin, I express gratitude. Gratitude for every culture, tradition, and person who fought for us to get to this point. Gratitude to have a tool to help unburden those so defeated by life that their day-to-day is a struggle. Gratitude that the mushrooms called out to me and showed me the path.

Should you become a facilitator or decide to partake in a psilocybin session, I encourage you to do a bit of inner digging to understand your intentions behind it. And perhaps give thanks to those who have been offering and using this medicine for centuries. Each person will have a different stance on this matter. But the only way to truly know how you feel is to process it out. Such contemplation will allow you to stand securely on your beliefs and give you a road map to move forward.

Colonization, Appropriation, and Capitalism

··················

If you would like to learn more about how colonization, appropriation, and capitalism have cast shadows over psychedelics, the Chacruna Institute is a leading resource on this topic. See their website (chacruna.net) for countless articles and books, including:

Psychedelic Justice: Toward a Diverse and Equitable Psychedelic Culture, edited by Beatriz Caiuby Labate and Clancy Cavnar

Plant Medicines, Healing, and Psychedelic Science: Cultural Perspectives, edited by Beatriz Caiuby Labate and Clancy Cavnar

Drug Policies and the Politics of Drugs in the Americas, edited by Beatriz Caiuby Labate, Clancy Cavnar, and Thiago Rodrigues

Women and Knowledge in Mesoamerica: From East L.A. to Anahuac by Paloma Martinez-Cruz

Summary

We must educate ourselves about the past in order to move forward in the right way. I believe it is important to respect the history of psilocybin, especially before you consider having a psychedelic experience. While it's tempting to jump on a plane to Jamaica or Peru for an all-inclusive resort psychedelic experience, there is a lot of homework I suggest you complete first. Giving thanks to the many cultures that have used this fungi ceremonially is important. Should you decide to try psilocybin, ensure your practitioner, therapist, guide, or sitter holds the space of respect and knowledge of this history. While we will never completely know the ultimate origin of this incredible fungi, we can trace its influence on the past and respectfully offer our gratitude for the opportunity to grow through its use in the future.

CHAPTER 4

The Effects of Psilocybin on the Brain

IN THIS CHAPTER, I will discuss the basics of how our brains function and what we understand about the effect psychedelics have on our brain chemistry. To be honest, the best that scientists have at present are theories. Sure, researchers have captured images of the brain while on psilocybin to determine which receptor sites are activated and such, but we do not yet know the whole story.

The human body has an intricate neuronal network with an incredible number of pathways running from the brain. The brain is made up of soft tissue that includes gray and white matter, non-neuronal cells, small blood vessels, and nerve cells. Non-neuronal cells help maintain the health of nerve cells and the brain, and blood vessels feed and oxygenate the brain environment. Using electrical impulses and chemical neurotransmitters, nerve cells—or neurons—send messages to different parts of the brain and the central nervous system, which then transmit those signals to other parts of the body.

Neurons communicate to the rest of the body about how to react to our environment, such as whether to move out of the way of an oncoming car, how to react to a stressor, when our blood sugar needs balancing, or when there's an itch to be scratched. A simple command to move may be conveyed with an electrical signal, whereas neurotransmitters communicate the need for more complex reactions, such as a change in hormones, a shift into sleep mode at night, or an elevation in mood.

A couple of neurotransmitters that you may be familiar with are dopamine, which regulates feelings of reward, and serotonin, which regulates feelings of happiness.

Let's look at an example of how dopamine works. I love Italian food, and my favorite dish is pasta carbonara. Every time I eat it, I simply feel *good*. When I go to my favorite Italian restaurant, the moment I see, smell, and taste pasta carbonara, dopamine is released in my brain. In that moment, I experience the immense pleasure I'm accustomed to. Another example comes when you repeat an activity that relaxes you or brings you joy. For me, it's walking in the woods. Every time I start a walk in our nearby woods, I am flooded with joy and a sense of well-being. Whether it's the colors, sights, smells, or a combination of them all, walking in the woods provides me with lasting positive benefits. For you it may be casting a fishing rod or clocking out of work. No matter the source, performing actions that release dopamine makes us feel good, so we crave to do them over and over. We want the repeated reward.

Serotonin is the neurotransmitter that has been studied most extensively in relation to psilocybin. Serotonin can elevate mood and make us feel happy, but it also contributes to sexual behavior, aggression, impulsivity, cognitive function, appetite, pain, thermoregulation, circadian rhythm, sleep, and memory. Although it functions as a key player in many biochemical, hormonal, physical, and emotional reactions in our day-to-day world, serotonin has mainly been researched for treating depression.

After ingestion, psilocybin converts to psilocin in the gut. Researchers have focused on how psilocin interacts with serotonin receptors in the brain. When we look at the chemical structures of psilocin and serotonin side by side, we can see that they are nearly identical. This resemblance allows psilocin to bind to serotonin receptors and thus elicit the same feelings of happiness and connectedness with the world.

Hallucinogens do not flood the brain with serotonin. Instead, they bind specifically with the serotonin 5-HT2A receptor, turning it on or activating it. (For those who want to go deep into the various types of serotonin receptors, of which there are fourteen, consider checking out the work of Thomas S. Ray.) Researchers are also investigating the various ways in which psilocybin may affect other serotonin receptors, potentially allowing for targeted use for specific mental issues such as PTSD, eating disorders, fear responses, anxiety, and addiction.

Psychoactive Drugs

A psychoactive drug is a chemical that changes the function of the nervous system and results in alterations in perception, mood, consciousness, cognition, or behavior. Psychoactives are consumed almost every day by almost everyone. It's true! The most common psychoactive substance in the world is caffeine, with alcohol at a close second. These chemicals quickly alter the brain and, in turn, how we interact with the world after their consumption. How many of you are one type of person before you drink coffee and another afterward?

There are four types of psychoactive drugs: depressants, stimulants, narcotics, and hallucinogens. These groups can be further classified as having nonaddictive or addictive potential. Depressants, stimulants, and narcotics have a high potential for addictive use. These substances affect a very specific part of the brain that stimulates the dopamine reward/reinforcement pathway and fortifies it. Think of it like an electrical current traveling down a line. Each time an addictive substance is used, neuron A lights up and signals neuron B, which signals neuron C, which releases the cascade of chemicals eliciting the "ahhhhh" reward sensation. Dopamine is the driving neurotransmitter in this pathway, and it is the quest for pleasure (or the escape from pain) that drives the brain to reinforce this pathway over and over. As with any neuronal pathway, the more you use it, the stronger it becomes and the harder it is to change.

The dopamine pathway isn't the only neuronal pathway that becomes hardwired. Most of our brain's neuronal pathways become somewhat cemented by the time we are teenagers. This occurs through learned behaviors, repetitive actions, and repeated experiences. Although this system is great in many ways, it can hinder our ability to grow and change when needed. Many years ago I began to see this hardwired system failing many of my patients, as the physical symptoms resulting from hardwired patterns were wreaking havoc in their lives. My objective as a naturopathic physician is to identify and treat the cause while soothing the symptoms. I needed to help my patients become aware of the automatic process of cause and effect that was happening inside them.

My patient Paul, for example, had chronic stress that resulted in heartburn, fatigue, increased sweating, and digestive upset. The cause of his stress was someone he had worked with for several years. Despite their contentious relationship, it was necessary for them to work together on many shared projects. The situation had gotten so bad that the thought of his coworker would cause the stress cascade to begin. I explained the neuronal pattern that had been established by his repetitive experience of working with this person. At this point, whenever Paul saw or thought of his coworker, neuron A would immediately light up and stimulate neuron B. Then neuron B would alert neuron C, and neuron C would elicit a number of physical reactions. The cascade turned on Paul's sympathetic nervous system at full throttle, leading his digestive system to shut down and his circulation and body temperature to increase. We had to shut this neuronal pathway down, and I suggested a neuronal repatterning approach.

Creating awareness within ourselves can be difficult, but it is not impossible. This approach requires immense concentration and patience. I suggested that when Paul saw, thought, or felt anything about his coworker, he should immediately start to concentrate on something else, something that he loved—his favorite place, an image that brought him joy, a positive scent or color. He needed to stop, freeze, and visualize in the moment. In theory, what this would accomplish would be that neuron A fires, but instead of the signal automatically heading toward neuron B it would be redirected by the image he loves to neuron D. When neuron A fires to neuron D, none of the neuron C physical reactions would be released and as a result Paul's burdensome symptoms would dissipate.

All of us adults have established an exorbitant number of automatic neuron pathways, many of which we aren't even aware of. Once on autopilot, these patterns can be extremely difficult to recognize—let alone shift—but I encourage you to consider all the possible autopilots you may be running on. The process of neuronal repatterning might be something worth considering as you begin to work with psilocybin.

The hallucinogenic group of psychoactives includes psilocybin, LSD, DMT, ayahuasca, synthetic mescaline, and peyote. While research indicates that these substances do not cause physical addiction, there is always a concern that they may lead to psychological addiction, or addiction to the experience. The use of hallucinogens does not lead to drug-seeking behaviors, and in my experience most users want and need time before considering taking them again. An integration period after use is common, in order to contemplate and process the experience. Psilocybin also has a built-in system for discouraging repetitive use, as a tolerance is built up quite quickly, diminishing its effects.

The Default Mode Network

As research and clinical trials have progressed, we've noticed that participants who take psilocybin have other, perhaps more noteworthy brain changes to consider. One such affected area is the default mode network. Most of us are familiar with the brain's regulation of the autonomic nervous system that controls our muscles and glands, our breathing, the beating of our hearts, and our digestive system. But there's another automatic system that is on all the time: the brain's default mode network, which includes the medial prefrontal cortex and the posterior cingulate cortex that connect via the angular gyrus.

The default mode network controls how we think and feel about things. It was once thought to only be activated in the wakeful rest or

PSILOCYBIN THERAPY ✦ 82

daydreaming state, but the default mode network has since been proven to be active during times of internal goal-oriented and conceptual cognitive tasks and when we are thinking about others, ourselves, the past, and the future. The default mode network may turn off when you're physically focused, as when you're playing sports, solving a complex problem with your hands/body, or meditating—when there is intense focus and concentration—but otherwise it is running its chattery thoughts continuously. How many times has a random thought jumped into your brain as you were reading this page? That's the default mode network at work.

As adults, our default mode network is firmly established, telling us how to react and feel about everything we come into contact with. Over the course of our early life, we built and established this default thinking through our experiences and exposure to the world (this is also where implicit biases are born). But when we are babies, none of those pathways yet exist. The neuronal highways at this point are wide open. As children our thoughts and actions sometimes go left, sometimes right, and sometimes in a circle. The element of surprise in the way young children move through the world is brilliant, and I wish we could all stay that open and use that much of our brains' potential forever.

Unfortunately, that isn't the case. Between the ages of six and twelve, we home in on a certain set of pathways, narrowing our potential to think outside the box. That box may be created by our parents, family, community, religious affiliations, teachers, peers—basically, anything and anyone outside ourselves. These developing pathways are influenced by our actions and the resulting rewards or punishments we receive, and they are reinforced repeatedly once they're established. At this point, it can be very hard to see, feel, think, or act beyond what we have created for ourselves. I know I'm making it sound like we become robots, but it can feel that way, especially when we notice our implicit biases or patterns in our lives that don't seem to match up with our authentic selves. And this is where psilocybin shines. Psilocybin offers the opportunity to rewire our neuronal pathways, because it has a profound effect on the default mode network.

A 2012 study performed at Imperial College London showed that when adults consume psilocybin, blood flow to the default mode network greatly decreased, in essence putting the network into a sedated state. Many people report a fear of taking psychedelics because they "will lose all control." As someone who struggles with control issues, I can whole-heartedly say that this is why I find psychedelics so healing. While our default mode network may be solidified as a preteen, that doesn't mean adults don't still have the capacity to construct different neuronal pathways with behavior modification. With the default mode network being turned down by psilocybin, so to speak, new pathways to think, feel, and interpret are opened more easily. The brain rises to the occasion, finding alternate ways to exchange and process information. By turning off that automatic thought and feeling machine, you are left to see things more honestly and often in more compassionate and loving ways.

Brain Waves

The neocortex is involved in higher order brain functions, such as sensory perception, cognition, motor commands, spatial reasoning, and language. Brain waves arise when a group of neurons in the brain send an electrical signal to another group. (This electrical activity is measured by an electroencephalogram, or EEG, and the machine's output is a series of waves.) Beta waves are involved in conscious thought and logical thinking and tend to have a stimulating effect, whereas alpha waves are produced when you are awake but not really concentrating on anything.

Measuring the brain waves of a person using psilocybin is another way scientists are studying its effects on the brain. The most noteworthy sign of psilocybin's influence is the marked switch from alpha-wave activity to a beta state, with a clear decrease in alpha waves and increase in beta waves in the neocortex. An increase in beta waves within the neocortex often leads to profound sensory experiences, mystical experiences, exploration of deeper feelings, and increased understanding and acceptance of oneself and the world.

Summary

We are barely at the beginning of our scientific pursuit to truly understand how psilocybin and other psychedelics affect the human body. While physiological research is valuable and fascinating, it may be that the subjective results of clinical research are more worthwhile. Talking with participants, listening to their experiences, seeking similarities, and understanding the long-range effects of psilocybin use may prove to be more valuable. Andy Letcher puts it perfectly in his book *Shroom: A Cultural History of the Magic Mushroom* when he notes that, despite all our scientific resources and research, we really can't fully comprehend what psilocybin does to our biochemistry. The best we can relate is that psilocybin is "the neurophysiological equivalent of turning over stones" in our brain to reveal new thoughts, insights, and feelings.

CHAPTER 5

The Role of a Facilitator

LET'S SHIFT OUR FOCUS NOW, turning toward an overview of what a psilocybin session is typically like in a Western medical model. When you begin to seek out psilocybin as a treatment option, it is common to have many questions, thoughts, and feelings. One of the best ways to navigate this new terrain is to take your time and find the right facilitator.

A facilitator is the person—a doctor, therapist, chaplain, nurse, sitter, shaman, curandera, healer, or guide—who determines the proper dosage of psilocybin, administers it, and sits with you during the session. The facilitator is there to offer support and ensure your safety. Choosing a facilitator is a personal decision, and I encourage you to give it some time and consideration. It's like finding a new doctor. In a broad sense, a facilitator should be someone you can be open and honest with in an environment of safety and trust. You are looking for someone who is qualified and who you connect with. Not every practitioner will meet the needs of every participant, so it is important to seek out a facilitator who understands you and can meet your specific needs.

In my opinion, a facilitator should be able to:

+ create a foundation of trust before, during, and after the session;

+ educate the participant about psilocybin, what they should expect on the day of the session, and what happens afterward;

+ remain mentally present during a session;

✦ gently support but never direct the participant during a session; and

✦ ensure the set and setting are well established.

Psilocybin opens you up in a very unique way. The facilitator is not there to tease out or share opinions about what a participant is doing, feeling, saying, or thinking during a session. Offering water if the participant sits up, taking notes of anything said, and offering periodic moments of support such as "How is everything going in there?" are all helpful. During the session, it is the participant's time to *feel*, not process through conversation. (Being a facilitator will require some shifts for those who are trained in traditional talk therapy.)

But there really is a lot more to consider. As more psilocybin facilitation centers open across the country, there will be a massive surge in the call for facilitators. Since a lot of us do not come from a ceremonial psilocybin lineage, we are being trained in a way that reflects the research practices of the last seventy years. Through this lens, regulating bodies have decided what skills and qualities are necessary for facilitators to qualify to practice. This model does not always consider traditional ways, and those who wish to use them may themselves jumping through regulatory hoops. Keep in mind that this is an emerging field, and it is changing almost daily.

In November 2020, voters in the state of Oregon passed Measure 109, which created a program for the administration of psilocybin products to individuals aged twenty-one and older. The passing of this measure paved the way for a two-year development phase during which an advisory board could discuss and formulate all aspects of the program, including manufacturing, training, and facilitating. Colorado recently followed suit in legalizing psilocybin for therapeutic use, and many other states are quickly coming on board. As you can imagine, as psilocybin therapy becomes legal in more states, there will likely be a lot of changes in facilitation and training.

Working with a facilitator with extensive knowledge of the physical, spiritual, and psychological effects of psilocybin is extremely important. From the perspective of the Western medical model, being skilled in these areas is just one aspect. The following should also be in the facilitator's wheelhouse:

+ use of a psychedelic harm reduction approach, in which a thorough conversation regarding both the risks and benefits of psychedelic substances is held with the participant;

+ best practices and up-to-date information regarding patient safety and knowledge regarding drug contraindications and patient medical history (Matthew W. Johnson and colleagues wrote the definitive compendium of safety procedures and ethical practices for psilocybin-assisted therapy[1]);

+ knowledge of key signs of medical and psychological adverse effects;

+ skills in managing or holding space for possible disorienting experiences of the participant, such as existential experiences, dissociation, disorientation, and loss of self;

+ in-depth knowledge of set and setting to promote the best possible outcome; and

+ subjective experience with psilocybin.

The current landscape of training for psychedelic facilitators is focused on a few programs. (For a list, see Psychedelic Therapy Training Programs in the back of this book or visit my website for up-to-date information.) Most programs require somewhere between 150 to 300 hours of training, which includes a combination of lectures, small-group discussions, reviews of therapy session recordings, mentoring experiences, and experiential and group learning. As the first state to approve

Protecting Traditional Facilitators

....

Throughout Mesoamerican history, curanderas were the facilitators of psilocybin through ceremony and ritual. Their intimate relationship with the mushrooms instilled incredible power and healing through psilocybin ritual.

As we move forward as a country, decriminalizing psychedelics and legalizing them into the Western medical model, we need to pause to consider not just the curanderas, but all other cultures and underground sitters who have been working in the ceremonious ways of psilocybin. These facilitators have repeatedly found themselves vulnerable to prosecution for such services and continue to be denied sanctity within the emerging profession. I encourage you to use your voice if you have had a positive experience with psilocybin and a facilitator of this type.

psilocybin administration in a medical model, Oregon has set forth a list of criteria that training programs must include. All programs, including those based outside of Oregon, must go through an application process to enable graduates to apply for a facilitator license, and potential facilitators also must take a state exam. You do not need to hold a professional degree. My guess is that as other states pass psilocybin such laws, they will put similar processes into place.

One question to consider is if you prefer a licensed facilitator or are comfortable with a facilitator who has not gone through institutionalized training but has gained skills and experience in other ways. You will find qualified facilitators on either side of that line.

How to Choose a Facilitator and Next Steps

Ideally, you would find a psilocybin facilitator through word of mouth. A referral from someone you know intimately that has worked in the psilocybin space typically is a referral you can trust. At this point, though, I'm afraid the next best option is researching and reading reviews online to determine who might be a good fit for you. Honestly, this sounds a little crazy to me, but without any type of psychedelic regulatory body, it will likely take a bit of trial and error. I encourage you not to skimp on your research; reach out and connect with the various organizations that have been present from the beginning. You can also visit my website for referrals and regularly updated information.

After making initial contact with a facilitator, you should have a short meeting to see if you connect enough to move forward with the process. If the facilitator feels like someone you want to continue with, then schedule a first pre-session. In the pre-session, the facilitator should lead you through a conversation to ensure you understand what psilocybin is, what it does, and the potential risks of using it. The goal is for you to leave fully informed and educated about what you are agreeing to do, as well as to begin building a relationship of trust with the facilitator. After the initial appointment, there may be one or two additional appointments before psilocybin usage is introduced.

These appointments are important because they allow you to continue to build confidence with the facilitator. Confidence will allow you to relax and release during your session, but it also creates trust that you will be safe during the experience. These meetings are the time to talk about your intentions, expectations, fears, and any other questions you have about the process. It's also the time to have clear conversations about touch—such as holding a hand, putting a hand on your shoulder, or a side-arm hug around the shoulders for support—so that you can set up comfortable boundaries and avoid alarm or confusion during the

Session Checklist

···············

✦ Find a reputable facilitator.

✦ Meet a few times beforehand to get to know the facilitator and discuss your intentions for the session. Ensure that you feel fully comfortable with the facilitator.

✦ Discuss what is and is not desired regarding touch during a session and create a plan for if that changes during the session.

✦ Consider the environment and whether you would feel more comfortable bringing a friend to sit out of sight to ensure your safety.

✦ Schedule integration sessions before the first session so they are already on the calendar.

session. (That being said, facilitators should always ask before initiating an agreed-upon touch during a session.)

The choice of reaffirming statements is another area to work on before your session. One of the biggest advantages of psilocybin is that it tends to bring to the surface what you need to look at. As humans, we have a natural tendency to run in the other direction when things arise that we don't want to feel or deal with, to push them away rather than face them. Psilocybin gives you fresh eyes and a different perspective from which to process old traumas, fears, and pain. Sometimes during a session there can be a moment of resistance as those feelings, thoughts, or memories arise. Reaffirming statements allow the facilitator to support your release of tension, confusion, resistance, or fear as you process these moments. Work with your facilitator beforehand to come up with a few statements to use as needed during the session.

Pre-session appointments are also the time for you to begin getting comfortable in the session space, getting familiar with the layout of the room and learning where the bathroom is. The art and decor should feel inclusionary and safe. The furniture should be placed in a way that makes you most comfortable. Don't be afraid to ask for something to be moved if it helps you relax. My colleague recently held a session where the participant requested that the furniture to be rearranged so that the facilitator's chair was not in between the participant and the door. Moving things around to ensure your comfort is easy to do.

The Qualities of a Good Facilitator

Janis Phelps, the founder of the Center for Psychedelic Therapy and Research at the California Institute of Integral Studies, wrote an in-depth piece on the role of a psychedelic facilitator called "Developing Guidelines and Competencies for the Training of Psychedelic Therapists."[2] In reflecting on this article, my education, and the facilitators I've worked with in my own sessions, I've summarized what I believe to be valuable skills and qualities for a facilitator. By no means is this list exhaustive, but you might want to look for these qualities when considering entering a relationship with a new facilitator.

Empathy

We must begin with empathy. In his landmark book *On Becoming a Person: A Therapist's View of Psychotherapy*, Carl R. Rogers referred to this attitude as unconditional positive regard. There should be no emotions or worth attached to what happens during a session. The facilitator should have a caring and unconditional regard toward the participant, and, whatever happens, the relationship is rooted in that foundation. Within a psychedelic session, the meaning of empathy stretches to also include a facilitator's ability to create confidence in the participant that they will be able to emotionally hold the space and the experience.

When working with participants who have experienced trauma, racism, marginalization, or cultural bias, a keen empathic ability is necessary. Participants are often vulnerable during a session, and having a skilled facilitator to hold your process—whatever that may be—in a supportive way is essential.

The best facilitator is one who can peacefully witness the participant's experience and calmly support only as needed. My professors often mentioned the need to train ourselves (especially those with a talk therapy background) in the art of "non-doing." With experience, a facilitator comes to know and trust that, whatever the session may be, their primary role is to provide a warm and caring attitude. Participants gain an intense awareness of their surroundings, which include the facilitator's tone, body language, and energy. If participants feel less than confident that their facilitator is kind, experienced, trustworthy, and there for them, the experience may take an unfortunate turn. The foundation of empathy is laid in the pre-session meetings and ideally should be firmly in place by session day.

The facilitator is there to create the type of space that will be of service to *you* and *your* experience. A facilitator should be actively and quietly present for you during the entirety of the session, with an open heart, a compassionate soul, and unconditional positive regard. To witness another's journey to this spiritual place is an honor, a gift that should be filled with presence, empathy, and gratitude.

Trust

Trust is another essential aspect of the facilitator-participant relationship. Without trust, it can be difficult for the participant to truly let go during a session. A foundation of trust should be laid well before the full session, and this is done through meeting, conversing, and preparing the participant. Although each and every session and participant is different, there are many consistencies across sessions that can be thoroughly discussed beforehand. Having this type of preparedness can ease the participant's mind, especially if they encounter a challenging moment or an emotional experience. Stan Grof, researcher and developer of holotropic breathwork, was very vocal regarding the importance of establishing self-trust within the participant, trust in the therapeutic relationship, and trust in the facilitator.[3] These aspects are all interconnected, working together during the session to strengthen the experience.

If, after meeting a facilitator, you feel that all your questions were answered and you feel safe in the environment and comfortable with the facilitator, that is a great first step! Continued interaction with your facilitator and learning the steps of preparedness should allow that trust to grow. Creating this level of trust allows the participant to be able to fully experience whatever comes during the session day with the knowledge that they are in good hands. Remember, there is no "right" way to be or act in a session, and most facilitators have seen it all. (Vomiting, bowel and bladder release, weeping, and extreme fear states are just a few of the more challenging aspects to some sessions.) You should be able to trust that whatever comes up for you—however beautiful or challenging—is what's supposed to happen and that your facilitator is there to support you. A good facilitator will not judge, allowing the participant to communicate moments of resistance or intense emotions (panic, fear, grief). This, in turn, helps the facilitator support you during the session. And, lastly, having trust in your facilitator lets you openly share your experience afterward, allowing you to integrate the session and hopefully bring more meaning into your life.

A few meetings before the session might not be enough time to develop your trust in a facilitator and move forward. Such hesitancy might be the result of uncertainty or fear of the unknown, but if it is because you are unsure if the facilitator is a good fit, then by all means change course. Having a trusting relationship in this type of work is truly necessary for creating the potential for deeply dynamic work, and the initial phases of building the relationship are an important part of the healing process.

Spiritual Intelligence

Through my travels and experiences, I've had moments of explicit feelings that could only be described as spiritual. Walking into The Miracle Church of Mosta in Malta, visiting St. Peter's Basilica in Rome, and standing on the top of Mt. Sinai in Egypt have created extraordinary feelings within me. It goes beyond wonder to an almost out-of-body sense of connection. Thoughts, feelings, and images rise to the consciousness, along with deep feelings of inner awe.

Having a facilitator with spiritual intelligence is of great benefit during a psilocybin session. Spiritual intelligence has been described as the ability to access higher meanings, values, abiding purposes, and unconscious aspects of the self and to embed these meanings, values, and purposes in living a richer and more creative life.[4] It is an understanding that all life on Earth is connected in some way, and therein lies the gratitude of interconnectedness. When we possess this level of self-awareness, it can greatly encourage transcendence, which Abraham Maslow defined as "the very highest and most inclusive or holistic levels of human consciousness, behaving and relating, as ends rather than means, to oneself, to significant others, to human beings in general, to other species, to nature, and to the cosmos."[5]

We really don't know what is happening when we have a psilocybin experience. How we will consistently think, feel, and process for the rest of our lives is essentially hardwired by age twelve. It almost seems inconceivable to me that there are ways in which I view the world at almost fifty years old that originated when I was a preteen. It feels unfair to be limited by something that I seem to have had no control over. But the blending of the two concepts of spiritual intelligence and scientific research elicits excitement in me. Spirit and spirituality are concepts, philosophies, and religious processes that perpetually ignite curiosities and often bring great meaning into our lives.

Having transcendent knowledge will allow a facilitator to be open and comfortable with whatever the participant may experience and share. Many psilocybin participants catapult into the realm of transcendence. Is this just a particular set of neurons firing in the brain, as seen on an MRI, or are participants tapping into the highest levels of consciousness? Either way, facilitators with spiritual intelligence are more likely to appreciate the realms of transcendence that a participant experiences and are better equipped to understand mystical consciousness.

A Sense of Humor

I've yet to meet a shaman, medicine person, or curandera who wasn't quite funny. A psilocybin session allows you to dive deeply into your healing process, but don't ignore the stops along the way that are showing you the humor in life. Being able to share these joyful moments with a facilitator allows for connection and a deepening of trust. When you find a facilitator with a sense of playfulness, you will find a welcoming quality that will support the lighter moments of your sessions.

Ethical Integrity

The importance of a facilitator who demonstrates self-awareness and ethical integrity cannot be overstated. Facilitators should be able to honestly identify their motives for doing this type of work. As a facilitator, I believe in the inherent healing ability of participants, meaning they know how to heal themselves. It can be easy for a facilitator to take on the role or persona of a healer, but in the Western medical model, the participant, together with the substance, are doing the healing. In talk therapy the therapist aids and guides the client in finding solutions, clarity, and behavioral modifications based on the conversations they share. In psilocybin therapy, however, it must be agreed upon that the facilitator is there to support the set and setting, ensure the participant's safety, and guide by doing nothing except supporting. By using psilocybin, participants acknowledge they will only find what they seek inside themselves. Therefore, dependency is placed on the participants' inner knowledge versus seeking answers, approval, or clarification from the facilitator.

PSILOCYBIN THERAPY ✦ 96

Because of the vulnerability that psilocybin often evokes, it is imperative that ethical integrity be at the forefront of every session. This is a big topic on a lot of our minds as we move toward legalization. At the time of writing, there is no regulating body for psychedelic facilitators. Luckily there are groups, such as the American Psychedelic Practitioners Association, that are diligently working to create platforms to uphold the highest ethical standards within the profession.

Beware of the Abuse of Power

When you are using psilocybin, you are permeable—meaning, whatever the facilitator does or says can have a big impact. As a participant, you should never feel disempowered by a facilitator. If you are not confident and comfortable, you may begin to question yourself or the experience. Participants need to believe in those who are guiding their psilocybin experience. They need to trust that the facilitator knows the process and how to hold space during a session. Distraction from this can greatly diminish the experience.

Power Differentials

Unfortunately, there is a history of abuse in the realms of medicine, therapy, religion, politics, and academia when actors have different degrees of power. Turning our view to psilocybin and other traditionally used substances, we must acknowledge that abuse has occurred here as well. Psilocybin takes us to a vulnerable place—ideally to have a safe and therapeutic experience. But there are people who thrive on power and knowingly (or unknowingly) utilize these substances to manipulate and harm those who partake in them. Though only a very small percentage, some facilitators do intentionally skew the experience during the vulnerable phase to exercise power and control over those they're entrusted with. I won't skirt around the issues that have arisen regarding some facilitators in their psychedelic practices. The stories are out there and, quite honestly, they are disturbing.

I want you to be informed about what is and isn't a part of a psilocybin session. My goal is to empower you so that you can confidently and enthusiastically use psilocybin for your healing needs.

At *no* point during a psilocybin session should a facilitator:

✦ demonstrate a power differential as authority;

✦ diminish your own power or confidence in the process;

✦ touch you in a sexual way;

✦ intentionally pull you away from your own thoughts and process; or

✦ force you into particular locations, behaviors, or thought patterns during a session.

When power dynamics play a part in healing, it is a red flag. I really can't be much clearer than that. This is an important time to trust your instincts. If you feel you are being manipulated or put in compromised situations or blatantly unsafe environments, you need to find safety. That can be in the form of another professional who is unaffiliated with your facilitator, a family member or friend, a chaplain, an online support group—really anyone who you can talk to. Having the opportunity to voice your concerns or questions, as difficult as it may be, could save you (and perhaps others) from harm and perhaps serious trauma.

A power differential occurs when a person interacting with someone in a position of authority is left feeling vulnerable. A common example is the power differential that can play out between medical doctor and patient. Many patients put their faith in the old adage that "doctor knows best." But without a proper balance of education, options, and teamwork between doctor and patient, it can leave patients in a vulnerable state. This differential plays out in our society in many ways, particularly among marginalized and BIPOC communities (Black, Indigenous, and people of color). Another relationship where power differentials can be witnessed is between therapist and patient. I have often had therapy sessions where I just wanted the therapist to tell me what to do or how to think about my life. Naturally this isn't the role of a therapist, and their doing so would have demonstrated authority over my life.

Because these types of roles are clearly marked by our society with labels such as *expert* or *leader*, it can be challenging not to assume they know best. Our society has also cultivated the notion that we are powerless beings who need a professional to make our health care choices for us. As a naturopath, I am committed to educating my patients, which often comes with a lot of room for listening as well. We are a team, but I rely on my patients to determine which treatment process they feel is best for them. Professionals, in general, should offer us help, education, and guidance that encourages us to find strength in ourselves and our decisions versus telling us what to do.

Another way to consider a power differential is when one person believes they have more power over the other and they act to assert that power. Again, we've seen this repeatedly throughout history in a myriad of ways, but it has especially affected BIPOC communities. The distrust, hurt, and surmounting damage members of the white race have placed upon BIPOC communities has the potential to create immense distrust between white facilitators and BIPOC participants. As I've repeatedly mentioned, trust and vulnerability are key points to any psilocybin session, and without them a session can be challenging or unfulfilling.

BIPOC facilitators are needed more than ever to work within their communities to create safe spaces for the natural emotional unfolding process to occur. The same goes for LGBTQIA+ communities and all marginalized peoples. Having facilitators with similar personal experiences and cultural backgrounds as participants can promote safety and understanding in psilocybin sessions. If you are interested in learning how to become a facilitator, check out the training programs listed at the end of this book or, by all means, reach out to me personally.

Unfortunately, although not prevalent, power differentials have been present in the psychedelic space. Our culture is obsessed with power, and many hurt and troubled souls seek to control others through powerful positions as a way to soothe themselves. Perhaps you have heard of the podcast *The Cut* and their segment on psychedelics. As the segment unfolds, you begin to realize that a darker side of psychedelic medicine has existed and that there are people out there creating strong power differentials with vulnerable participants through the use of these substances. I share this to bring awareness. The majority of facilitators in the field are working diligently to relieve suffering, not cause it. Psilocybin and other psychedelics have an immense potential to heal, but we begin to wade into deep traumatic waters if our sessions are not led with trust, an open heart, and the highest of integrity.

Transference and Countertransference

We've all done it. We meet someone at a gathering who reminds us of someone else and, no matter how hard we try, we begin to transfer our old thoughts about the person we once knew onto the new individual. This, in a nutshell, is transference.

In the psychedelic space, transference occurs when a participant transfers thoughts or feelings about someone in their life onto the facilitator. When empathy, compassion, grief, or anger are present in a session, the participant will sometimes transfer those emotions onto the facilitator. This can be a helpful experience when the facilitator acknowledges the transference and is not triggered by the reactions, instead offering gratitude and appreciation for the participant expressing themselves. In my MDMA training sessions with MAPS, we repeatedly witnessed transference during sessions and, amazingly, the facilitator's kind words of appreciation in return.

It isn't easy to have a participant yell at you in anger during a session. But receiving a participant's emotions with compassion and grace, no matter what they are, has an incredible effect. Participants are almost puzzled by the response of gratitude, as if they were programmed to brace themselves for the response they were accustomed to: rejection, aggression, demoralizing comments, nothing. When they don't receive the response they are used to, their brain and body must respond differently. This is the way in which transference can be used therapeutically during the psychedelic session and, with reflection, during integration sessions to heal.

When transference isn't helpful is when the facilitator gets triggered by what the participant communicates. Reacting in a negative or overly personalized way toward the participant derails the session. For example, if a participant speaks to a facilitator in a way that reminds the facilitator of her abusive father, she might be triggered into a defensive response. But a skilled and experienced facilitator knows how to properly hold space for the participant and that the session should always remain focused on the participant's experience and potential healing.

Countertransference is the flipside. Countertransference is when the facilitator transfers feelings to the participant. Having a strong awareness of and ability to recognize transference and countertransference is important for any facilitator. Countertransference often results in the facilitator moving the boundary of separation between themself and the participant. It can result in disclosing personal information or dispensing advice in place of therapeutic listening. An overt countertransference is when there is a sexual attraction to a participant. While sexual attraction is not an issue per se (we are all human, after all), *acting* on those feelings is. It is imperative that the facilitator be able to identify what is happening and have the ability to make appropriate changes or remove themself from the therapeutic relationship as needed to eliminate harm.

Professional Background

When you begin your search for psilocybin sessions, you will see facilitators with various backgrounds. Is one better than the other? Is one more skilled or safer? Maybe. It's about finding a facilitator with the skills and qualities I shared above. The right facilitator will be determined by you, not the letters behind their name. Here I'll provide a quick review of the most common professions of those engaging in this work, so you can better understand their skill sets.

Therapists

Eliciting meaningful conversations with participants before a session can result in more productive outcomes, but uncovering a participant's intention for a session is not as easy as it sounds. While there are many gifted individuals with a natural knack for such matters, a trained therapist can cultivate incredibly meaningful conversations. Psychotherapists and counselors typically earn a bachelor's degree and move onto a master's degree, or they may earn a doctorate. All of these professions have extensive training and knowledge in the mental health arena, but that is just one aspect of the psychedelic space.

Health Care Professionals

As a naturopath I was trained to treat the whole person, meaning that I look beyond the symptoms. Frequently in my private practice, I encounter patients whose illness is a direct result of an imbalance in their mental state. Most commonly it was anxiety or depression stemming from trauma or feeling as if they were locked into life choices they had made.

Naturopaths are trained as Western medical doctors with an additional 300 hours in traditional medicine therapies. We are trained from the start to build relationships with our patients, and we do this through active listening and education.

Other types of health professionals who are emerging as psilocybin facilitators include medical doctors (MDs), osteopathic doctors (DOs), nurses, chiropractors, massage therapists, and energy workers.

Clergy and Religious Leaders

Clergy are the formal leaders within an established religion. As many people seek solace in their relationship with spirit, their shaman, rabbi, pastor, minister, or priest are natural facilitators for their communities.

Sitters

Sitters are those with psychedelic experience who can be with you during a session to ensure both physical and emotional safety. They can come from almost any type of background. As with any type of facilitator, their role is to support you through the experience: to hold your hand, offer you water, and support you should more challenging aspects arise. Although there are psychedelic sitter programs across the country, many sitters are self-taught or have found their path through using these substances.

Perhaps a friend or family member asked them if they would sit for them. That is how one sitter I interviewed came to realize where his skills and passions aligned. After his first session as a sitter, a great sense of gratitude came upon him. He talked about how witnessing another dislodge the inner critic was an honor. His own experience with psilocybin had shown him the "wow" of life, and helping facilitate that for another was immensely gratifying. Educating himself and offering to sit for others created the experiential foundation of his work. When I asked him if he believed that there should be formalized training, he paused. He felt that while there are good and not-so-good things that come out of regulation, the fact is that instituting regulations will inhibit some people from participating. His greatest concern, though, was how to ensure safety and accountability within the sitter community.

Traditional Ceremony

Ceremonial use follows the traditions of indigenous use. These practices vary from origin point to origin point, but often include any combination of fasting, purifying, fire, music, dancing, prayer, meditation, spiritual bathing, and solitude. The shaman, chief, curandera, witch, healer, doctor, or other traditionally labeled person guides the ceremony and its purpose.

Solo Sessions

I recently read a thread on social media regarding one man's solo psychedelic session. The only reason he did it by himself was because he couldn't find anyone to sit for him. Based on his description, it seems he might have had a more enriching experience if he'd had someone there to support him. But where do you start? Since psychedelic sessions aren't currently legal in most of the world, how do you find someone to assist you on the journey? You may consider asking a friend, preferably one who has had personal experience using psychedelics so they know what to expect and how to support you.

Dr. Bill Richards is an extraordinary researcher who has dedicated his life to psychedelics and the mystic consciousness. As a young man, he went to study in Germany and happened upon a psychedelic research trial about retrieving early childhood memories that needed participants. He was curious to try psilocybin, and the experience ultimately put him on a trajectory he could never have imagined.

Later, as he was preparing to leave Germany to return to the United States, he asked the study supervisor, Dr. Hanscarl Leuner, who by this point knew him well, if he could participate in one last session before he returned home. Leuner obliged but told Richards he was too busy to sit with him and that he would need to find someone else to do it. So, he grabbed the only other English-speaking student he knew and proceeded with the session. But this session was like none he'd had before. He became profoundly paranoid and fearful of his surroundings and the people in it. The poor sitter, having had no experience with psychedelics or therapy, was of no help. Thankfully, Richard's prior experience with psilocybin allowed him to pull himself through.

My advice is this: don't carry out your first psilocybin session alone or with someone who doesn't have experience in altered states.

Summary

A facilitator, although not typically long term, is often one of the most profound relationships you will experience in your life. Together you can safely navigate an experience that can only be described as ineffable and life-changing. I have witnessed incredible facilitators skillfully support deeply traumatized participants safely through sessions that have transformed them on almost every level. These relationships are not to be decided on spontaneously or on a whim, but should be considered and planned with intention. If you do so, I've no doubt you will be led to the right facilitator.

CHAPTER 6

The Session

AS WITH MANY THINGS IN LIFE, there's often a mixture of emotions when we consider exploring new territory in a psilocybin session. We are more able to take risks when we're younger without all of the mental roadblocks we develop as adults. As I've gotten older, it has become harder and harder to venture outside of my comfort zone. While my life has been dedicated to self-growth and the journey, as I've aged, fear and uncertainty sometimes cloud my visibility into new directions. I've also learned firsthand that not all self-growth experiences are particularly pleasant. There have been a few in my past that have felt like a cold, hard slap in the face. When you consider taking psilocybin for the first time, it will undoubtedly bring various thoughts and feelings to the surface. Some of them may be founded on the persistent messaging you grew up with that all psychedelics are bad, but many others—such as fear of losing control or of walking into the unknown—can also come up.

Later in this chapter I'll share the flow of a typical session under the Western medical model, but it is important to know that there are many different ways to experience psilocybin. No matter whether you proceed traditionally or via our developed Western way, honoring the past, the lineage, and the sacredness of the altered state is most important.

Some of you may be able to relate to a first-time psychedelic experiment with friends in your youth—often an unbridled experience crusading into a new world. Research has shown that we don't fully realize all the potential consequences of our behavior in our youth. Social settings are still a common environment for psilocybin adventures and can create positive shared moments between friends such as taking psychedelic mushrooms together during a full moon, on a camping trip, or in the safety of a friend's house. But is being with others always the best way to get what you hope for from psychedelics? Healing can occur in social settings, but in these environments, it is often spontaneous rather than intentional. When we enter this type of work—using psilocybin with a focused intention—we are tuning in to an intentional healing space.

To direct your intention toward healing, a psilocybin session will typically have the best outcome if it is free of distractions and social engagement. This allows you to feel safe to go inward and have an intense personal experience. Where we start shifting away from the social experience is where the term *set* is rooted. Part of the meaning of *set* in this context is the intention behind why you are taking the psilocybin as well as your mental state. Your facilitator will guide you through conversations to better understand what the intention of your session will be.

Please don't misunderstand me here. As psychedelics enter the mainstream, there is a focus on using these substances to heal and connect. I'm not saying you cannot have profound and extremely personal psychedelic experiences in a social setting—as I believe you can—but from personal experience, my witnessing, and research from countless participants, I believe an eyes-closed, no-distraction session consistently correlates with deeper experiences of healing and an increased chance of mystical interaction.

The contextual setting of historical Mesoamerican psilocybin ritual use includes symbolic, social, cultural, psychological, aesthetic, and musical elements.[1] While *set* and *setting* are modern terms in the context of psychedelic space, it is clear that the lineage holders of psilocybin strongly believe in the value of being present with the space, the participants, and the substances throughout the ritual. Researcher Ido Hartogsohn recognizes that our Western definitions of set and setting are too limiting. Traditionally, he noted, the inclusion of music, symbolism, religion, and ritual played a much greater role than the comfortable room that is the setting of the Western model. Lineage holders who have used psilocybin in ceremony for generations formed a relationship with its use that curated the set and setting in a way that was inclusive of their culture.

Alfred Matthew Hubbard, otherwise known as "the Johnny Appleseed of LSD," witnessed this level of devotion to psychedelic rituals while visiting Mexico. He observed that the ritual use, songs that were sung, and varying ceremonial aspects impacted the participant as well as the facilitator. Upon returning home, Hubbard cultivated the terms *set*, referring to the participant's mindset, attitudes, and beliefs, and *setting*, meaning the physical and social environment of the session, and encouraged their use in the research space. The concepts of set and setting were implemented in clinical trials as early as 1958 as one type of control for the studies. Over time, Hubbard developed rooms that were more conducive to relaxation and an overall feeling of peace. The patients reported feeling more comfortable in these rooms, as they were less clinical and more like a home setting.

As I move the conversation regarding set and setting forward, I recommend a few best practices we should consider adopting for the Western model. There is a difference between a traditional ceremony space with a lineage holder and the criteria developed for the Western medical model. Read on to get a firm grasp on how best to incorporate set and setting as a support for yourself and your session.

The Set

In Western psychedelic research, set refers to the mindsets of the participant and the facilitator. It's important for you to be in a good headspace going into a session and for the facilitator to be fully embodied. You want to be reasonably distanced from recent emotional events such as the death of someone close, the recent loss of a job, or the ending of a relationship. While psilocybin can help in times such as these, it's best to have some space between the actual event and a session to avoid the session getting thwarted.

In the early years of psychedelic research, there was some experimentation with how different sets affected patients. For example, changing a clinician or staff member's attitude from warm and friendly to cold and impersonal produced a higher probability of unpleasant effects for the participant during a session. Not preparing a first-time participant about what to expect in a session also contributed to negative experiences. Repeating these set experiments proved time and time again the importance of the set in achieving a more enriching and positive psychedelic experience. Research has also shown that participants have keen insight into the mood and emotions of the facilitator during sessions. While increased empathy is a reliable outcome of psilocybin use, one might consider the possibility of it also increasing clairsentience.

It's vital to spend some time thinking about the session beforehand. Sharing your questions, concerns, and fears with the facilitator during pre-session meetings helps create a positive set. Becoming familiar with the session space and talking through the natural progression and timeline of what the experience will be like is also helpful. But in my opinion, the best set preparation you can do is to acknowledge and hold the notion that you are entering a safe and sacred space. Do so with gratitude for those who came before you and go with an open heart.

The Setting

Setting refers to the space or environment where a psilocybin session occurs. In traditional ceremonies, sessions are held in someone's home or in a sacred space. In the Western therapeutic model, the setting is in a hospital, theraputic space or clinical setting. Sitters tend to work in spaces they have created for sessions or in your own home, and a large contingency of people feel they can only do psilocybin if they are outside.

The setting also refers to your comfort level with the facilitator, for without an ability to relax and let go you will likely get stuck from moving into and through the experience. Creating the set and setting are important aspects of being a facilitator. The session space must be comfortable and aesthetically pleasing, and the decor should feel inclusionary and safe. Ideally there is a bathroom in the session room so you don't need to leave the sanctity of that space. Eyeshades, headphones, and several music playlists are typically available.

Another thing I suggest, as will most facilitators, is that you bring a few items to personalize the space for yourself. This can include photos, art, or something of comfort. You may end up never looking at these items during your session, but I find them to be more helpful than not, especially toward the end as you are transitioning back to the conscious mind state, when personal items can be helpful to contemplate.

Remember, part of the process is choosing the setting that feels the most comfortable and safe for you.

Psilocybin Dosage

It takes some experience to determine dosage for a psilocybin session. Traditional psilocybin lineage holders receive the dosage via spirit guides and the mushroom spirits themselves. The sitters I interviewed mostly agreed that there is a level of intuition involved in determining dosage but that pre-session conversations were often the best indicators. Western facilitators, on the other hand, follow regulated dosages for the therapeutic model.

Since the 1950s researchers have used a synthesized psilocybin dose between 20 and 30 mg, which seems to be the best amount to achieve feelings of unity, self-love, and mystic consciousness. Lower dosages have a tendency to not cross the desired threshold. When the dosage is too low, the opportunity to quiet the default mode network is greatly diminished and the participant often remains in the conscious mind. This can be a disappointing and frustrating experience.

But what about higher doses? Researchers have reported that participants who have taken 4 to 10 times the amount of psilocybin often do not experience the positive effects of self-love or feeling connected with oneself and the world around them, instead reporting overwhelming sensory input of visuals and feelings. Without having the ability to relate to what we felt afterward or process what we thought, scientists see little value in administering high doses. This is why for most first-timers the typical dose will generally fall between 20 and 30 mg of a synthetic psilocybin or 2 to 3 grams of dried, whole psilocybin mushroom. This equivalent is the clinical standard today.

I have my own thoughts on higher doses and do believe they hold value for highly skilled psychonauts, but such journeys are for those who are highly invested in the field of mystic consciousness and altered reality. Heroic doses (the name given to large psilocybin doses) have provided many people with a unique insight into thoughts, feelings, and visions outside of normal reality. A well-experienced participant who has used psilocybin with regularity may begin to get curious about signs or symbols that they have consistently experienced during sessions. In the beautiful book *Wound Swimming: Healing with Psilocybin, Ceremonies and Microdosing* by Tiana Griego, she shares her experience with taking higher doses but only after she built a relationship with psilocybin to better understand it. As she puts it, the sessions with larger doses help her to encode something that is very unique to her existence. She looks for repeating symbols and keys and has been piecing together knowledge that is specific to her. Griego is a member of the Creek Tribe, Indigenous Mexican, Dutch, and Welsh; perhaps the higher dosages are allowing her to tap into ancestral knowledge.

Oregon, the first U.S. state to legalize psilocybin therapy, has created a foundation for the therapeutic model that includes the use of whole dried *Psilocybe* mushrooms rather than synthesized psilocybin. In the Western model, the mushrooms will most likely be delivered via capsules at the start of the session, but other psilocybin facilitators have their personal preferences for delivery methods. Some will offer

Disclaimer

....

The author and editors of this material have made extensive efforts to ensure that treatments and dosage regimens are accurate and conform to the standards accepted at the time of publication. However, constant changes in information resulting from ongoing research and clinical experience, reasonable differences in opinion among authorities, unique aspects of individual clinical situations, and the possibility of human error in preparing such an extensive text require that the reader exercise individual judgment when making a clinical decision and, if necessary, consult and compare information from other sources.

participants the whole dried mushroom to chew and swallow, while others like to make a tea from ground psilocybin. Others finely grind the mushroom and add it to chocolate. The standard research dosage of synthetic psilocybin in the therapeutic model is 20 to 30 mg, and sometimes a booster dose is given around the one-hour mark.

The Attendants

A facilitated session is a psilocybin session with a participant and a facilitator. A one-on-one facilitated session is one participant and one facilitator. A one-on-two session can either be one participant and two facilitators (the common research model) or it can be one participant, one facilitator, and one ally.

The facilitator is the one who ensures everything is unfolding as it should to promote and protect the participant and their experience. An ally is someone the participant knows and trusts who is willing to come and simply hold space. An ally should typically remain out of sight.

Allies can bring comfort to participants, especially when it is their first session or they need more assurance of their safety.

An ally is not necessary in most situations, but should you feel better by having one, discuss it with your facilitator. When choosing an ally, ask yourself:

Can you relax into the experience with that person in the room?

Will they neither distract nor make you feel self-conscious?

Do you trust them and feel they have your best interest in mind?

Can they sit for four to six hours quietly?

If so, then they are probably a good ally for you.

Music

Music can play a big part in a psilocybin session. If chosen well, it can support the natural unfolding of the process. If not chosen well, it can distract and return you to a more conscious state of being.

Sound is embedded in the psychedelic space from its tribal and cultural history. Songs, chanting, the beating of drums, and so much more can be found when we look to the original users of psychedelics. The music often helped initiate the participant into the experience and then took them on the journey, depending on what was played, sung, and chanted and when. This sonic landscape created a sort of slow climb to the peak of the experience and then a gentle decline. Psychedelic researchers have mimicked this approach and created playlists to guide the participant in much the same way. (For a list of some of these music playlists, see "Psychedelic Music Playlists" in the back of this book.)

What is the best type of music to play during a session? As long as it is not a playlist of songs you know, you'll be ok. When you recognize a song, your conscious awareness can click on, causing you to rise up from the deep dive of more important work you might have been doing.

Many facilitators suggest that music without lyrics, ambient nature sounds, classical music, and chanting are all good choices. Another consideration is silence, which many people prefer. Music should be an accompaniment to a session, not a distraction. If this area interests you, consider exploring it further. As we move into this new era of psychedelic use, musicians and enthusiasts are bringing this type of work into the fold.

The Use of Eyeshades and Headphones

Eyeshades obviously turn off one of our biggest sensory organs, the eyes. Sight stimulates an immense amount of neuronal activity in the brain; by reducing that input, you are decluttering the psilocybin experience. Sight is also processed in a way that typically utilizes our conscious mind. When the eyes are given a break, it can support the process of deeper connectivity.

Should you not like eyeshades or headphones, take them off. Remember, this is *your* journey. You may enjoy silence or the natural sounds going on around you. You may prefer to set your gaze on an object or image, and that's ok. Keep in mind the facilitator has a dual role: to support your process and to encourage you to relax into any resistance that arises. If the reason you want to take off the eyeshades or headphones is because in doing so you can break away from a part of the experience you don't want, the facilitator might encourage you to do your best to stay in the experience. If wearing either or both of them is inhibiting you from going deeper into the experience, then by all means communicate that to the facilitator.

Other Things to Have on Hand

While the facilitator should provide music, a comfortable space to lay down, blankets, headphones, and eyeshades, there are some things that you may want to bring with you on session day. Basic comforts like a water bottle and perhaps a piece of fruit or small snack for after the session are nice to have on hand. While some participants prefer not to drink or eat during or immediately after a session, some do, and having a snack available is helpful. Eating typically brings you out of your psychedelic experience, as it turns on the digestive process, so I suggest waiting until you are ready to resurface before eating.

I always recommend wearing extremely comfortable clothes on session day. Sweatpants, cozy sweaters, fuzzy socks—whatever makes you relax into comfort, wear it.

Another tip from my teacher, Dr. Bill Richards, is to bring something to look at immediately after taking the psilocybin. On average, it takes between thirty and fifty minutes before you can feel the effects. It's helpful to have something inspiring or contemplative to look at, like a nature book with large photos or art that inspires you—anything that can promote relaxation of your mind and body can help you go deeper into your experience. You can also consider bringing photos of loved ones. These can serve as a grounding point to bring you comfort and peace, if needed.

Another common item to have in the room is flowers, particularly roses. According to Maria Mangini, writer, nurse, and psychedelic leader, the rose has a long history of importance in many cultures, including the Sumerians, Egyptians, Chinese, and Greeks. Thirteenth-century poet Rumi said, "Come out here, where the roses have opened. Let soul and world meet." Sometimes participants say they can dive into a rose, or dive into mystical consciousness from looking at one.

Richards often mentions the tradition of the rose and its part in psychedelic research since early studies in Saskatchewan on the treatment of alcoholism. When study participants emerged and took their eyeshades off during a session, they would intuitively let their gaze rest on the rose, which would seem to unfold and open before them.

The Session

When session day arrives, there will be a mix of emotions, especially if it is your first time. Try not to dwell on them too much. Simply observe what you are experiencing, perhaps journal, and then move forward. If there are feelings of hesitation or an intuitive feeling that it isn't a *safe* situation, however, please take a step back and reconsider. Trust yourself. You can always come back to the experience.

You will most likely begin your session in the morning. There are several reasons for this. One is that a typical session is four to six hours long. Beginning in the morning allows you time to integrate back into a normal state and get a good night's sleep afterward. Another reason is that psilocybin is best taken on an empty or almost empty stomach. Beginning in the morning means no fasting is required over the course of the day. Personally, I like beginning in the morning because it reduces the anxiousness of waiting all day. If a session is set to start in the afternoon or evening, I tend to overthink throughout the day.

You should be made to feel comfortable once you arrive at the setting, ideally a space you've visited before for your pre-session appointments. This is the time to settle in and create your space. You and the facilitator are now moving into a space that should be solely focused on you. This is your day, your experience, and your space for the time being. The facilitator may ask you to set out anything you brought so that it is easily within reach should you or the facilitator need it. The facilitator will take some time to check in with you as well, asking how you are feeling and if you have any questions or want to go over anything before you begin. This is the time to reiterate instructions and review agreements regarding touch, intention, and affirmations.

After you feel you've covered all that you need, you'll be given a psilocybin dose in one of its various forms. If given the dried mushroom form, you'll be asked to chew it up before swallowing. I find that if I macerate the dried mushroom for a long time, chewing it down to a pulp, it decreases my chance of stomach upset.

Using the *Tibetan Book of the Dead* as a Guide

....

In 1964, in the height of the psychedelic awakening in the United States, Timothy Leary, Ralph Metzner, and Richard Alpert published *The Psychedelic Experience: A Manual Based on the Tibetan Book of the Dead*. The volume was meant for anyone experimenting with psychedelics who wanted to learn more about how the *Tibetan Book of the Dead* could be used as a framework to guide one through a psychedelic experience.

In the simplest of terms, the *Tibetan Book of the Dead* was created to guide the recently deceased soul on its journey from life to death. The Tibetan name of the book, *Bardo Thodol*, can be translated as "Liberation Through Hearing During the Intermediate State." Tibetan Buddhists believe that the soul, upon leaving the physical body, would begin its journey through the confrontation of life, both the good and the not-so-good. This journey played out with the presentation of pleasant or wrathful deities to demonstrate one's life choices. As you can imagine, this may be hard to witness or even frightening. The *Bardo Thodol* was created as a comforting tool, to be read aloud to the recently departed soul by a brother monk to explain to the soul what it was encountering in an effort to calm and ease its journey.

Leary, Metzner, and Alpert saw this journey as one that mirrored a psychedelic experience. Their goal was to help those using psychedelics better understand where they are in the journey so they can continue along the path. The goal is to reach liberation during a session, to let go, relax, and receive the experience.

The first phase of the journey, the chikhai bardo, can be compared to the first phase of a psilocybin session. We come into the awe-inspiring phase, when ultimate truths are revealed and conscious-expanding experiences are had. This first phase can last only minutes if you are clinging to control or hours if you allow the experience to open up within you. Leary notes that anyone who hasn't had proper preparation or who desperately clings to their ego may find this phase difficult, especially if they don't have much experience in tranquil meditative states. This is the time to relax into what you may experience. You may see and feel things that relate to your life or that seem outside of yourself. It is an interesting transition point where you almost forget that you've moved into something not completely conscious.

During the next phase, called chonyid bardo, unusual thoughts, visions, or hallucinations may occur. The brain is now randomly pulling files. If you can resist the need to find meaning or organization and simply watch them go by, these thoughts and visions can produce meaningful results later. The most important aspect of this phase is to relax and let what is being experienced move through you. For me, this is the part of the experience when I lose all sense of time. I'm often deep diving in between meaningful thoughts and images and random ones. For example, in one of my sessions I remember experiencing the pain of a past relationship. I then witnessed the release of that pain and the release of it holding me back through a series of images. Afterward, it swiftly morphed into a comforting forest scene. These types of images, oscillating between recognition and abstract, can be quite common during this phase of the session.

The final phase is sidpa bardo, the period of quiet reentry as you try to regain your ego and normal mental state. You'll rise up to consciousness and slip back down into the experience less and less. Don't rush, just relax and let it play out completely. Even if a session has been challenging, if it is closed with a gentle sidpa bardo, you will typically experience an integration of positive reflection. One session comes to mind when I think about sidpa bardo. I worked with a client who experienced quite a difficult session, with a lot of fear and at times panic as she worked through past trauma. Despite it being a more difficult session, once she reached the sidpa, she was calm and incredibly centered. She later recalled that this time in the session was the most powerful as she had walked through the fear and made it to the other side, feeling stronger than ever.

Learning about the *Tibetan Book of the Dead* before a session is one way to prepare so that you have tools to navigate any potential distress or distractions. In pre-session conversations with your facilitator, you can talk about the phases of the *Bardo Thodol,* creating opportunities for them to give you reminders or refocus points during a session to move you toward liberation.

After taking the dose, it's time to relax and wait. Pull out that big picture book and flip through the pages. I find this type of tool helpful, as trying to create small talk during this waiting time can be challenging for some. During the waiting period, some facilitators may offer craniosacral massage or reiki, light touch energetic techniques that can create a smooth transition from the normal to the psychedelic state.

After a little while, it is usually a natural transition to want to lay back, put on the eyeshades and headphones, and go into the experience. Simply observe and feel what is happening. Do your best not to judge, try to understand, or assign conscious thought to the experience. Processing is best saved for afterward during integration sessions.

The only job of a participant is feeling. Truly! If you can stay with what you are feeling instead of trying to assign meaning, there is greater potential for deeper connection, understanding, and healing. Sometimes there are moments during a session when you want to understand why something is happening or coming into your field of thought. But when you allow yourself to rise back up to the surface of consciousness, you lose the deeper experience that the psilocybin creates. We all have incredible power to pull ourselves back to mental awareness, but if you stay within the deeper states of the subconscious during your session, it typically proves to be a more enriching experience. If you notice yourself rising to the surface of consciousness, do your best to relax back into the session. Your facilitator may offer a simple suggestion to help you dive back in.

As the psilocybin starts to work, you may feel like talking or remaining silent. Either is fine, but if you need to express or share your thoughts, do so. At any time during your session, should a negative or anxious repetitive thought arise, please tell your facilitator. These stuck thoughts, if verbalized, seem to know how to move out of the way. Facilitators are trained and have experience in helping to clear these thoughts to allow for a deeper experience.

Sometimes you will have that initial flash of clear light, ego dissolution, or entheogenic experience only to suddenly resurface relatively soon after. You may notice a glimpse of ego or routine reality return. The ego is not as it once was and you may feel caught in between paradigms. You may wonder, "Am I dead? Who am I?" It can be challenging if you are attempting to understand what's happening from your routine reality because that reality isn't fully there. Try to push away distractions. Perhaps focus on someone or something that brings the feeling of enlightenment to you (Buddha, Christ, the forest, Einstein, the ocean, Lao Tzu).

Anxiety can arise, but this is a transitory phase. If you notice uncomfortable physical feelings, your facilitator is with you and will remind you that you are safe. To help you stay within the feeling part of the experience, the facilitator will listen and offer appropriate responses, but they most likely will not push the conversation. This is the time to ease back and witness what is happening for yourself.

A wide range of possible physical symptoms can arise with psilocybin. As the session progresses you may notice a slight increase in your heart rate or clammy hands. You may feel the need to yawn or have a slightly excitable sympathetic state. Trembling or a sense of heaviness are also commonly reported. It can be difficult, but if you can identify these troublesome symptoms as precursors to a transcendent experience, perhaps you can shift your conscienceness away from them. Try to gently meditate and remember that releasing, trusting, and going into the experience will move you toward liberation.

Nausea can often be reduced or eliminated by ingesting the mushrooms on an empty stomach or with just a bit of something like plain toast; some people prefer eating whole mushrooms with peanut butter. Brewing the mushrooms into a drinkable tea also helps to reduce nausea. The psychonauts of the psychedelic world believe that nausea is the spirit moving around and is the first sign of the magic mushroom working. Leaning into that sensation can often eliminate the nausea, but either way, it is typically a short-lived symptom.

Sometimes people need to purge at the beginning of a session, which can include vomiting, diarrhea, or spitting. If purging needs to happen during the session, your facilitator will not judge you but instead support you through it. Purging isn't a sign of failure or that the psilocybin is not working correctly. In many indigenous traditions, purging is a part of the process and is considered a cleaning out phase. Once the purging is over, the participant can relax onto the couch or bed to ease into the session. As an herbalist, I know plants that purge our bodies have a place in healing. While Lobelia (*Lobelia inflata*) is more modernly classified as an emetic, it was traditionally used to purge and purify the body. People often felt stronger after taking it and an increased sense of well-being from the intense purging it caused.

You may find that you have to use the bathroom, which is not a problem. Just let your facilitator know. Ideally there is a private bathroom within the space, so you don't have to leave the safety of the room during the experience. Ask your facilitator to assist you to the bathroom, as walking may not be as easy as you think. The door may not have a lock, which is simply to ensure you do not accidentally get locked in the bathroom during the session. While I'm a big believer in the universe's sense of humor, I think I'd prefer a comfy couch and blanket to the bathroom floor.

Rising to the Peak of Experience

As you move closer to the peak of the session, you'll begin to sink deeper and deeper into the intrapersonal experience. You may lose your sense of time and space as you float to the conscious realm less and less. This is the time to trust yourself. As the psilocybin takes effect, things will arise in your psychedelic consciousness. You may relive experiences of your life and feel them deeply. With your eyes closed, you may have visions that include imagery, events, geometric designs, shapes, patterns, and colors. Some people report feeling colors or seeing sound. Whatever is happening for you is your journey, and you should trust that the experience is safe.

Once you feel or recognize the shift away from consciousness, you'll want to try to remain within it as long as possible. You may feel bodily sensations or slip into a sleep-like state where time and space are no longer relevant. You may be beyond words, space, time, and a sense of self. Relax into it and go with what you are experiencing. The two things you don't want to do at this point are rationalizing what you are experiencing or trying to control what is happening. This will only shorten your time in this incredibly powerful state.

As your experience progresses, your facilitator may meditate, stretch, journal, or just sit. I adopted Ralph Metzner's term, alert quietism, for this state. Keep in mind that facilitators are humans with human needs, so they may excuse themselves to go to the bathroom but will always be close by.

All manifestations that arise during this phase of the session are manifestations from your own brain. Let me say this again, because it bears repeating: all visions and thoughts that arise during this part of the session are manifestations from your own brain. This can be difficult for participants to embrace, because what arises can range from joyous and funny to curious to angry, sad, or fearful. Those with a history of trauma may cling to their standard control mechanisms as to not allow that part of them to die. When something arises that elicits fear

Plant Spirits, Archetypes, and Symbols in Altered States

....

Throughout the centuries, many people have reported visions of Queen Toloache after the ingestion of sacred datura (*Datura wrightii*) and of Teonanacatl and the Bee Man while using ayahuasca and psilocybin, respectively. Guanyin, Shakti, Buddha, and Jesus are common archetypes participants report seeing in psychedelic sessions. Others report experiences where they are with ancestors or find themselves in a time in the past, before their own lifetimes, conducting healings or witnessing events. These types of experiences are labeled as hallucinations, but I believe they are real representations and not simply inventions of the mind.

In addition to such shared visions, seasoned psilocybin users may see the same image repeatedly over several sessions. Perhaps such visions have something to do with our relationships to archetypes or symbols in our ordinary lives. Having signs and symbols that we identify with or recognize in a session may be one way for our brain to accept and process information. For example, Guanyin, the goddess of compassion, appeared in one of my sessions. Having studied Chinese medicine, I knew of her and had often felt drawn to her image.

or grief, we have a natural tendency to look or run away from it. When something you don't want to see shows up in a psilocybin session, you may try to resist it by rising to consciousness, taking off your eyeshades and headphones, sitting up, or engaging with the facilitator. These tactics cause you to disengage from what the psilocybin is trying to help you with. Tell your facilitator and try to utilize your reaffirming statements to settle back and trust in the process.

Spirals and geometric patterns are very common visuals to experience during psychedelic use. (To get an idea of what these types of visuals may look like, check out the work of artist Alex Grey.) Many people have drawn the images they've seen afterward only to reveal exact replicas of Paleolithic cave drawings. So what does it mean when multiple people report seeing the same thing? Dr. David E. Nichols of Purdue University stated that these patterns might be similar among participants due to the specific effects of psychedelics on the brain. South African archaeologist David Lewis-Williams has studied this subject and believes our optic system generates consistent shapes during altered states, which gives rise to similar experiences. In simple terms, because our physical brains are similar, we all see similar patterns.

Another theory is that we are acting as a receiver of universal information once our default mode network is turned off. Or perhaps we are conditioned by our psychological experiences, culture, religion, and education. But that isn't how I have experienced it. For me, James Fadiman explains these shared visions best: "If you're comfortable with the notion that plants have intelligence and are part of the habitat of other intelligences, then [the idea of shared consciousness] is common sense. But if you are still committed to the notion that the only kind of intelligence is like ours in some way, you will feel that the question has not been at all answered."

Staying with a visualization can help you move into and feel whatever it is you are experiencing. I once worked with a participant who loved the ocean. She felt very comfortable in the ocean waves, even when she tumbled in the crashing surf. She had the glorious ability to relax in those moments and let the ocean take her to the surface. This was a powerful tool for her during uncomfortable moments in her session. If she felt resistance to what she was experiencing, she could return to her beloved ocean and remember the feeling of relaxing into the turbulence.

By standing still, taking a breath, and relaxing back into the experience, you might be surprised by the truth of what you reveal to yourself. I won't say that if you walk through the fire, every psilocybin realization is an epiphany of joy. But participants consistently report that—no matter what they experienced in a session, even when it was unexpected or challenging—the lessons learned were nonetheless extremely valuable. So, if a giant serpent appears to you during a session, don't run away. In Mayan culture, serpents represent rebirth and renewal. Walk willingly into its mouth to see what it has to show you.

The Comedown

The effects of psilocybin typically last for four to six hours, depending on the dose. At the end of your session, you may notice yourself rising up to consciousness and going back down for shorter periods as the psilocybin leaves your body. This is a normal experience. Others may feel that they are deep within their session until all of a sudden they return to a normal state. Using photographs, flowers, a fire in a firepit, or other tools at this point often helps with the transition.

Familiar patterns of thought and perception of the environment return. Most participants feel dreamy or fuzzy at this point. Some will have no hunger at all, whereas others may desire a piece of fresh fruit for nourishment. (Be aware, though, that eating and the digestion process will swiftly pull you out of the psychedelic state.) Do not rush this phase. Both you and the facilitator need to feel confident that you are ready to end the session and move out of the space. For obvious reasons, participants should never drive themselves home. In the pre-session appointments, you should discuss who will be your contact person to drive you home and get you settled for the night.

The most important thing at this point is for you to have time to yourself. That doesn't necessarily mean you need to be alone, but you need the time and space to do what feels best for you. Some participants

Bad Trips

As Terence McKenna used to say, "There are no bad trips." This term often refers to a participant feeling as though they are losing their mind, feeling deeply afraid, or almost anything that poses great challenges during a psychedelic experience. In naturopathic medicine, we use the term *healing crisis* when a treatment causes rapid healing that initially brings discomfort to the patient. It happens so fast that symptoms can often appear to worsen and then quickly shift to great improvement. While symptoms can feel intense and uncomfortable, they often lead to significant healing. When I think of bad trips, it reminds me of a healing crisis.

McKenna thought that a so-called bad trip reflected participants' overwhelm from having to learn faster than they were accustomed to. If your brain is suddenly flooded with new thoughts, patterns, and connections, it could easily create distress. But keep in mind that psilocybin simply shows us what is below the surface of our consciousness. To some, this may be shocking. Again, having a good facilitator and the proper set and setting will allow you to work through these difficult periods.

I spoke with preferred being alone in nature to sit and think. Others had a strong desire to be with family and express the gratitude they received from the session. If possible, do not return to normal life for the rest of the day or the next. You still may not feel like eating for hours after your session, which is ok, but I would suggest staying hydrated. Don't try to process mentally at this point, just relax and stay suspended in the experience. Rest, meditate, and sleep. Take time during the following day to begin to integrate your experience. Working, household chores, or parenting separate you from the opportunity to think, feel, and question what you experienced in your session. Get out your journal and write down what you remember of your experience. This may help your future integration sessions with your facilitator.

After the Session

Once you've returned home, you may feel tired, quiet, jubilant, dazed—any number of things that will be unique to you. What you've just experienced will most likely be incomprehensible at this time, so I recommend not trying to understand it right away. My first recommendation is to check in with yourself. Do you need to rest or hydrate? If you are hungry then eat what you'd like (consider having this prepared ahead of time). Give yourself plenty of time and space to just *be*. Let the thoughts come and go as you recalibrate to normalcy.

Over the next few days and weeks, you'll begin to process and integrate. Make this a gentle process without any pressure to figure it all out too quickly. There have been times when my processing took months for me to understand. Everyone is on their own timeline. Sometimes the epiphanies you experience during a session make you want to create big changes in your life. That is okay, but my advice is to integrate fully before making any big shifts. Sometimes we think a message received during a session means one thing but it turns out to be something else entirely after integration. Keeping connected to the process through journaling, therapy, meditation, exercise, or however you choose is a good practice.

Summary

A therapeutic psilocybin session is grounded in the preparedness of the participant. Finding a good facilitator to guide this process is just one aspect. Understanding your intentions, the set, and the setting are all of equal importance. This careful consideration will hopefully build your confidence in the therapeutic process. Remember that the session and the environment in which you conduct it should provide ample room for you to safely experience whatever arises. Utilize your reaffirmation statements in times of turbulence, and trust that your session will play out exactly how it is supposed to. Embrace the journey and allow the rose to unfold within you.

CHAPTER 7

Integration

INTEGRATION IS THE PROCESS OF UNDERSTANDING all the parts of ourselves in order to reunite them back into the whole. This includes the parts that arose during your psilocybin session. Integration is a big topic of discussion within the Western medical model of psilocybin therapy. Perhaps it's because the emerging model is mirroring the clinical trials that got us to the legalization point, or it may be due to the fact that so many involved come from a therapy background. Either way, when it comes to psilocybin therapy most practitioners believe integration is key to the healing process.

Working through life's experiences with the assistance of psilocybin can require some pretty heavy psychological lifting. The layers that tend to reveal themselves in a session can be surprising and sometimes complicated to navigate. I've completed sessions where I felt that nothing I experienced had particular meaning, only to later attend integration and have a world of new understanding dawn on me. A skilled integrator can help turn your psilocybin experience into a journey of curiosity and self-discovery. These new insights can create powerful shifts in how we view ourselves, our world, and our place within it. It can be very easy for me to turn a blind eye to internal pain or self-identifications that are not in my best interest. Having someone to help me draw those pieces of myself into the light can be difficult, but I'm always grateful and happier for having done it.

Another way to look at integration therapy is like a shirt that has several holes cut out of it for one reason or another. This shirt is a part of us, and trauma or certain experiences can remove pieces of it, creating holes. Integration involves looking at the holes with curiosity and beginning to understand why they were cut out. With integration therapy, once we reach a place of understanding we can sew them back onto the shirt, reuniting them with their whole. This reflection can be likened to shadow work, which I'll get into more a bit later in this book.

The initial pre-session appointments with a facilitator build the foundation for safely exploring new territory as it arises, both in the session and afterward during integration. While a session is uniquely your own, having a facilitator check in and make notes regarding the things you share or vocalize during a session is extremely valuable. These notes are pearls to return to afterward, helping to jog your memory and allowing for deeper process work. Even if you were silent the entire session—which does happen sometimes—there may still be a need for integration therapy afterward.

From my personal experience, the more opportunities I have to talk about a session, the more meaningful it can become, especially when unfolding experiences around trauma—hence the need for a safe and solid relationship between facilitator and participant. The first integration session is usually a time to recount the session and try to make some sense of it all. There may have been a pivotal part of the session that triggered a trauma response, whether it be a memory or reliving an experience. This first integration session is an opportunity to mentally work through these thoughts and feelings and begin to process the experience.

Working through thoughts, feelings, mental images, and emotions of a psychedelic session can be overwhelming and can take time, which is why having more than one integration session is recommended. When someone says one psilocybin session is like ten years of talk therapy, they aren't exaggerating. A lot can suddenly surface that needs to be worked through. One facilitator I spoke with provided a good visual to consider: when you have a session, you often reach into yourself and pull out a pile of potentially useful material to work through in integration therapy. This is also the reason why spacing out psychedelic sessions might be best, to give the participant an opportunity to work through the current set of issues before unearthing more. For veterans suffering from PTSD, for example, three psilocybin sessions spaced one to two months apart, each followed by several integration sessions, has proven extremely effective.

Although it's possible to do this integration work on your own, it can be difficult. Working with someone experienced typically achieves greater integration. We humans have the most incredible way of not seeing the whole picture. Here's an apt analogy that someone shared with me: Imagine seeing a stranger running from your neighbor's house with their puppy. You look at your neighbor's house and see their front window has been smashed. From your perspective, someone is stealing a puppy from your neighbor. But what you couldn't see from your perspective is the fire that broke out in the living room of the house. That stranger walking by caught sight of it and the puppy scratching at the window to get out, so they threw a rock at the window and ran down the street with the puppy to go get help. I share this story because we often only see the person running down the street. When it comes to our own lives, we often have huge blinders that limit us to our subjective and personal perspective. To actually turn and see the fire can be very difficult, especially if the fire is the trauma of our lives.

The last psychedelic session I had was with a seasoned sitter. I was contemplating joining an established team of facilitators and felt it important to get the feeling of the space while in a session. I wanted to ensure I could feel safe and that the space accommodated a participant's needs, and I wanted to experience being held in the session space by the facilitator to ensure that our values aligned. I had been meditating on my intentions for the session beforehand and kept returning to the same theme: is the facilitator role right for me?

The session, surprisingly, triggered a deeper internal process than I expected, and it was actually quite a playful one. I went in deep, rarely surfacing or having much I wanted to converse about. While it was a joyous session filled with immense gratitude, there was a lot that I went

PSILOCYBIN THERAPY ✦ 130

through, including some deep release of past trauma. I did my best to write everything down in my journal afterward, but I still felt there were big parts to potentially process and integrate that I had missed. Unfortunately, I wasn't given the chance to integrate with the sitter afterward, as that wasn't something he offered, which left me with a lot of heavy lifting to attempt on my own. Luckily, I connected with a seasoned integration therapist, who helped me process the thoughts and feelings that had arisen, clear the confusion, and better understand the experience.

Accessing Integration Therapy

Integration therapy can look like many things, but it typically falls into one of the following models: within a clinical trial, with a mental health facilitator, with a separate integration therapist who your facilitator has a relationship with, or with your sitter.

In the last couple of decades, the only legally available psychedelic sessions were through FDA-approved clinical trials being run through Johns Hopkins University, MAPS, and in clinics around the country. The Heffter Research Institute is another powerhouse for psychedelic research, having funded more than two-thirds of the psychedelic trials conducted to date. A clinical trial is a good place to begin if you live in a state that has yet to legalize psilocybin treatment.

The protocol of most clinical psilocybin trials goes as follows. Each candidate is screened and undergoes an initial interview. If approved for the study, the participant and clinical team then have two or three pre-session appointments. After each of three psilocybin sessions, typically conducted with two facilitators present, the participant has two or three integrative sessions with a member of the clinical team.

Although clinical trials are the most widely available legal option, there are some issues to consider before deciding to participate in one. First, clinical trials require a large time and energy commitment. What if you have your first psychedelic session but don't want to do the second and third? Another important consideration is setting up for a smooth transition out of the study. Most participants bond with facilitators after such deep work, and it can be emotionally difficult to sever that relationship. Experiencing a life-changing session only to be cut off from the research facilitators who supported you can have its own set of negative outcomes. Therefore, having an integration therapist outside of the trial is important for most participants to feel fully supported. On the plus side, however, facilitators involved in these clinical trials are some of the most experienced in the world, and their skill at conducting integration sessions is often what creates lifelong gratitude in participants. Clinical trials can be a great place to begin treatment with psilocybin, as they are often a low-cost option with highly skilled professionals.

As we begin to move forward with legalized psychedelic sessions, you'll be able to work with a state-licensed facilitator. Choosing a facilitator with mental health experience can be particularly helpful to those with PTSD or a history of physical or emotional trauma or addiction. Such facilitators include doctors, nurses, counselors, psychologists, therapists, and psychiatrists. Many of these professionals have already facilitated psilocybin sessions underground, and their professional background is extremely valuable in the integration sessions afterward.

Another choice is to find an integration therapist, who might work in tandem with a facilitator or separately. Either way, ensuring that they have personal experience with psychedelics is recommended. It can be a challenge to discuss psychedelic experience with your regular therapist if they are naïve to such experiences. Ensuring you feel understood without judgment is crucial when sharing your thoughts, feelings, and experiences after a psilocybin session.

Types of Therapy That Can Be Helpful for Integration

Integration can create meaning from your session experiences. It helps you process the things you thought, saw, and felt during your session to bring understanding to your life. This meaning can be achieved by working through specific trauma, behaviors, or life obstacles. But how do you do that exactly? Integration can be accomplished through cognitive behavioral therapy (CBT), transpersonal therapy, internal family systems (IFS) therapy, eye movement desensitization and reprocessing (EMDR), and somatic work. Integrative therapy incorporates a variety of techniques, but these are the ones I have an affinity for and whose effectiveness I've personally witnessed.

Cognitive Behavioral Therapy

Cognitive behavioral therapy is a type of talk therapy that works to connect thoughts, feelings, and behaviors. The first step in CBT is to develop an awareness of when certain thoughts arise, how they make you feel, and the behaviors that result from them. Creating awareness can be done through dedication and practice. Using CBT to help tease out thoughts and feelings that arose during a psychedelic session can lead to great insights. Taking this process one step further, acceptance and commitment therapy (ACT) teaches you to release control of the thoughts and feelings and to simply accept them and yourself as is.

Transpersonal Therapy

Transpersonal therapy, another CBT method, is extremely valuable for those who have mystical experience or transcendence during a psychedelic session. An integrative therapist with this type of background will easily be able to meet you when sharing your experience. They will often have knowledge of various religions, cultures, and archetypes and can aid in teasing out the meaning of certain images or experiences that occurred during your session.

Internal Family Systems Therapy

Psychologist Richard C. Schwartz developed internal family systems therapy after years of private practice. Schwartz continually had his patients talk about their inner lives and the conflicted parts of themselves that lived there. We all have aspects of our inner lives that we like and ones we don't like. IFS therapy can be helpful when trying to better understand why we place protective barriers in our mental consciousness. Although these barriers serve a purpose, protecting us from mental suffering and hurt, they remain long past the trauma and affect our lives in complicated ways. There are also parts of us that may do things that general society views as wrong or bad. Often we hide these parts of ourselves behind lock and key for fear they might be seen.

Eye Movement Desensitization and Reprocessing

This type of psychotherapy enables people to heal from the symptoms and emotional distress of complex trauma. EMDR is a useful tool to disconnect traumatic memories from the thoughts, feelings, and physical symptoms that arise when they are remembered. These events are considered "unprocessed," and by working through them in conjunction with rapid eye movement patterns, the patient teases apart the event/memory and the resulting thoughts, feelings, and physical sensations. This creates room to process the trauma.

Somatic Work

Receiving massage, reiki, craniosacral therapy, or other energy work can be particularly valuable for those who experienced a lot of energy moving or becoming stuck within the body during psilocybin sessions. Connecting our mind and body can produce profound results, and gentle touch can elicit key insights into the experiences felt during sessions.

Summary

My two cents? Find a facilitator who offers integration after the session or find an integration therapist with subjective psychedelic experience, especially if it is your first time. Share your experience, thoughts, and feelings—even if they sound crazy or you have no idea what they mean. An experienced integration therapist can help you navigate your experience through your personal lens without judgment. In processing your session, great healing and peace can happen. There is no such thing as too much support for the first go-around.

CHAPTER 8

Welcome to Your Shadow

WHEN I FIRST HEARD OF SHADOW WORK, I had all sorts of ideas about what it meant. In shadow work, we examine our behavioral and emotional terrain. The process draws on psychological concepts commonly based in Jungian therapy and is used to explore the parts of ourselves that we consider undesirable.

Some think of the shadow as the dark side of your personality, the part you hide from others to ensure the safety of acceptance in the hope of being loved. Many people have been conditioned to think of anger, frustration, confrontation, depression, and anxiety as bad. Whether due to our experiences, societal beliefs, upbringing, or religion, many of us efficiently hide these emotions away.

But I believe the shadow is much more than the emotions we look down upon. As we move through life and all its experiences—early friendships, going to school, romantic relationships, the ever-present influences of marketing and the media—we are constantly receiving messages from the outside world about what we should like and not like about ourselves. Those seemingly unlikable parts of ourselves can get pushed down into the shadow realm.

Over time I've gained a multifaceted view of myself. There's what I intuitively know to be true about myself (my authentic self), what I know has been curated to fit into society, and the part that still has a lot of work to do. The last part is not only the self awakening to conditioned bias but a whole mixed bowl of soup that tends to not serve my highest self.

In my youth, I was particularly judged and ridiculed for my choices. The way I thought and how I expressed myself just didn't seem to ever work in my favor. My thoughts were abstract, wild, and risky compared to the norm. On the outside, I looked like most white Midwestern kids in the 1970s and 1980s. My life consisted of school, friends, swimming in the summer, and a lot of TV. But when I was about seven years old, I noticed a change in how people reacted around me. I remember a deep sense of feeling misunderstood so often that I began to stop talking, realizing it was much safer to just observe. At times I'd slip and blurt something out, only to be quickly reminded that my opinions were *off* in some way. This feeling of isolation created a lot of negative self-talk— I'd tell myself I was stupid, immature, not worthy. The need to constantly pivot to produce a socially acceptable version of myself was very exhausting.

This dichotomy—feeling one way on the inside, while believing I needed to play the role of another person for the outside world—gave me stomachaches and eventually led to depression. I was so blinded by my old pain, masked in conflict with all my different selves, that I was rarely aware of what I was saying or how I was presenting myself to the world. While this started a pattern that produced a lot of wrong turns in my life, it also instilled in me a desperate curiosity to figure out what the hell I was doing because it *felt* all wrong. I wanted to understand why I always felt conflicted and surrounded by people who didn't understand me, when a huge part of me on the inside just wanted to be free like a horse running in the wild.

As unique individuals with separate and distinct paths, we humans are all susceptible to physical and emotional trauma. Some of that trauma is easy to identify, as it is overt and socially labeled as such (Think sexual/physical abuse, PTSD etc.). Our behaviors as children sometimes elicit such strong responses from our parents and caregivers that we learn quite quickly not to repeat them, especially when those behaviors lead to physical or verbal abuse. We do our best to avoid any type of behavior that leads to punishment. Those behaviors get stuffed way down, and we only adopt those that will keep us out of harm's way. But there is also a world of trauma that goes unseen or isn't considered "bad enough" to be called trauma, even though that's what it is. We receive normalized messaging that minimizes our traumatic experience. When the cues given to us as children tell us to be quiet, be good, or fit in, or when we are told there is something wrong with us, we take it to heart. When a child takes a risk and is rejected, it sends a clear message not to take that risk that again.

I've spoken with so many patients who had no idea that what they described to me was, in fact, trauma. As a society we've decided to categorize human experiences and put them into neat little boxes. If what you experienced doesn't fit into one of those boxes, it isn't worthy of being considered trauma. The truth is, if the experience continues to affect you, it most likely was traumatic and the process of turning towards it, let alone taking it head on, is a brave commitment.

Healing, learning, and growing is a lifelong process. The way you eat, sleep, and exercise will ebb and flow as you make your way toward health, slowly and steadily. You will start, do well, slip up, stop, and start again. Emotional healing is much the same. There will be times when you have incredible leaps in understanding, epiphanies even. You'll ride on these new feelings based on breakthroughs made, and your life will shift. But don't be alarmed if you slip. Triggers are buried deep within us, and they can show up in a multitude of different ways—even when we think we've healed. Something you thought you had processed can return so intensely at times that you may feel great sadness, frustration, or grief.

Working with your therapist, family, minister, or friends to tease out the trigger will be easier as you grow in your self-understanding. You'll have greater clarity in understanding why the trigger arose and set you off. This alone can bring comfort, as you move out of the unawareness phase of emotional chaos and suffering. But you must recognize that this is just a resting point, a place to work through what has come up and process it into your emotional understanding. After some time, it is almost inevitable that you will come to another mountain to climb, another hurdle to cross so that your growth can continue. You will be asked to make a choice: stay on the plateau or continue to climb.

Carl Jung said, "Until you make the unconscious conscious, it will direct your life and you will call it fate." If we can open up to the possibilities of what that means, maybe we can shift our lives in a positive way. What unconscious junk have we accumulated and how is it playing out in our daily lives? How did the shadow get created? And what determined which aspects of ourselves got to stay and which parts were hidden away? The shadow encompasses all parts of ourselves that we've learned to not express. It is our environment that dictates which parts to keep and which to stash away. But stashing these parts away doesn't remove them from our being. They are still there, tethered, waiting to be reunited with the rest of us.

The creation of the shadow begins soon after birth. As newborn babies, we are all perfect. We each arrive with thousands of unique qualities within us in just the right combination that makes us who we are. It's only once we're exposed to other people that we start to question ourselves and our self-expressions. Our earliest interactions are with our parents or caretakers. It is these interactions that can shift which parts of ourselves we show to the world. As toddlers, we are taught the rules through our environment and the consequences given should those rules be broken. We naturally strive for love and acceptance in life; through the experiences we have as young children, we begin to shed those behaviors that don't bring us closer to that goal.

There's more to what we stuff away than so-called bad expressions, though. For example, my son came into this world ready to do everything himself. At times this created a lot of frustration for both me and for him, as we had very different perspectives on what we were trying to accomplish. I was often just trying to get out the door, while he was creating independence and developing skills within the safe confines of our home. Getting his own coat and shoes on was a regular example. After noticing my repeated frustration while he was attempting to do this, he began to stop trying. My insensitivity and focus on getting out the door made his ready-to-try independent attitude get stuffed away because he didn't like the reaction it caused. While I wasn't intentionally hurting my child, I was hurting him nonetheless.

When I envision the shadow, it makes me think of a backpack full of all the parts of ourselves that we were told were no good and the messaging attached to them: "I can't do anything right." "I'm stupid." "Don't speak up." This backpack can get stuffed with so many parts that, by the time we reach adulthood, it can really be weighing us down. Because it's on our back, we rarely see it; because it's filled with parts of ourselves, which never actually detach, it is impossible to take off. The idea of opening the backpack to look inside may sound quite scary at first. But if you can remember that what is inside the backpack is you, and all parts of you are valuable, maybe it will give you the courage to try. This is a peek into your shadow. (You can see a video on my website that provides a great visual for this concept.)

Psychedelics are one way in which we can safely explore our shadow self to better understand our full selves, the patterns in our lives, and the suffering which is on the wash-and-repeat cycle. Psychedelics can provide us with an opportunity to move past the protector part of our trauma in order to see it with fresh eyes. According to IFS therapy, a *protector* is created when we experience trauma in our life. The protector guards us from feeling pain or emotions attributed to fear, anger, grief, vulnerability, or sadness and affects how we react to stress, interact with others, and think about ourselves. Like the fight-or-flight theory of trauma, which relates to the overproduction of cortisol with repetitive stress, the protector loses the ability to recognize when trauma is no longer present and it keeps us stuck in the trauma-reaction phase. Some experiences are so painful that the creation of the protector is necessary for survival, making it particularly difficult to shift certain behaviors in an ordinary state of consciousness. Psychedelics can allow us to seek out and dismantle the protector and discover what is on the other side of it.

I recently went through the MAPS MDMA training with Michael and Annie Mithoefer. It was an extreme and powerful experience to witness participants being guided through the MDMA sessions. These types of sessions can be raw, intense, and often healing. The ruptures that are created within our emotional terrain from trauma can be far and wide. It's as if the earth is cracked open and there is no way to cross from one side to another. Where you stand there is a protector warning you of the dangers. Sometimes the protector whispers the dangers of crossing in your ear, but at other times it yells in your face to stay away or tries to physically restrain you. The protector will do whatever it takes to keep you safe. If you get too close to trying to cross, the protector mentally moves you to safety far, far away. It may tell you stories to evoke fear. What needs to be so vitally shielded that the protector won't let us see? Typically, it is a fractured self, a memory or series of experiences that were so painful that our protector decided enough was enough. Unfortunately, this protection inhibits our ability to see and interact with these parts of ourselves. And because those parts go unseen and unprocessed, they often have an impact on our emotions and behavior.

Psychedelic therapy bridges the gap between consciousness and subconscious trauma patterns. It is one way to approach the trauma, opening a gateway to ease suffering by allowing us to embrace the parts of ourselves we've rejected and hold them with compassion. In a supportive environment with experienced facilitators, making the journey toward trauma can be manageable. The empathy of the facilitator combined with the empathy-producing substances make shadow work possible. Psilocybin and MDMA turn on self-compassion, unity, and empathy, granting us the opportunity to explore the landmines of our emotional terrain. Even after years of refusing to look at the despised parts of ourselves that we consistently reject, psychedelics can help us identify those parts, better understand why we disregarded them, and find the compassion to accept that they are just as important as the parts we love. Having the experience of self-empathy can be life-changing. Psychedelic therapy can help make our fractured selves whole again.

Cultural and Lineage Trauma

....

Psilocybin and other psychedelics are also used with a focus or intention on ancestral lineage healing. These practitioners believe that the traumatic events our ancestors experienced are embedded within our emotional DNA and that they can be healed through us during the present time. Healing the past through ourselves may seem far-fetched to some of you. As someone who has participated in this type of work, though, I found it to be transformative.

With the assistance of psilocybin, participants have been able to work through familial lineage trauma, often resulting in feelings of release, calm, and peace within. This work can bring up a lot of mixed emotions, so having a facilitator that can hold understanding and compassion for your lineage is important. During sessions, participants have also encountered ancestors who impart insights. In fact, it's quite common to encounter ancestors, archetypes, gods, and goddesses from various traditions while in a session. They all represent an opportunity for inner healing in deep and meaningful ways through your own subjective interpretation. Trust what is coming through.

The Inner Healer

When working with psychedelics, I often get asked "What is going to come up during my session?" Another way to put this is, "Which trauma is going to show itself?" The answer is that no one knows. This can be alarming for most people with no psychedelic experience. While we are all wanting to heal, being prepared for healing is something altogether different. According to Dr. Bill Richards, if a person is ready to work through a particular trauma in one's life, it will typically rise to the surface during a session. But if the participant isn't quite ready, the trauma usually won't present itself.

In Western psychedelic therapy, the inner healer is often discussed as the main driving force of what one will experience in a session, and it's what most Western-trained facilitators are drawing upon during a psilocybin session. This inner healer lives on the other side of the protector. I often refer to it with my naturopathic patients as well. The Western medical model has conditioned us to rely on a doctor to tell us what to do, what to take, or how to fix our body. At some point along the way, we traded our own healing knowledge for the all-knowing power of a medical model. Medical advancements are much appreciated, but it is important to keep some of the patient's inner healer knowledge and abilities in the mix.

After a new patient consultation, I tend to ask the patient to tell me in their words what *they* think is going on. Giving their inner healer a chance to speak has proven valuable more times than not. By tuning in to their inner healer, we often start off in the right direction instead of running through my endless list of tests and possible diagnoses. Teaching, encouraging, and trusting the inner healer is of great benefit in trauma work. You know yourself better than anyone and, as a facilitator, I'm here to encourage you to remember that.

Psychedelic substances are a way of encouraging your innate inner healer. The facilitator's responsibility is to support you safely toward where *you* are going by encouraging you to try to stay in emotionally uncomfortable places and to feel and go into any discomforts in your physical body. We also remind you of your inner healer and ask you to share what it is saying, if you're able. This is how you navigate your journey and find your way to the ruptures of your life. Then, your inner healer can begin to share with you the truths about your pain so that you can see it clearly—perhaps for the first time in your life.

Facing our shadow, the darkest parts of ourselves that we've so diligently tucked away for no one to see, is big, *hard* work. Even in the best of set and settings, we can experience challenges and sometimes there will be heavier than normal emotional lifting. When we are being blocked from moving forward in a session, sometimes the cause can be pinpointed and sometimes it cannot. This is where an experienced guide is invaluable, offering suggestions to help you call upon your inner healer. If the block or resistance continues, it can cause a physical distraction as an attempt to stop the progression toward emotional revelation.

Here is one example of a block. Peter had suffered on and off from depression, anxiety, and melancholy for years. He wanted to better understand why this had plagued his life, as he had no memory of what he referred to as "intense trauma." During his second psilocybin session, he quickly became uncomfortable and was unable to relax into his experience. His conscience turned on physical symptoms that dominated his entire experience. For Peter, it was an unbearable heat rising in his body. Although his blood pressure, temperature, and pulse were normal, he could not find relief and all thoughts were focused on that singular thing—the heat he felt in his body—what I call a block tactic.

Ideally, as facilitators, we have the right thing to say or do to help the participant turn the corner from this physical distraction. But sometimes the block is there for a reason, and the participant isn't ready. Although blocks can be extremely frustrating for the participant, this is when we must honor and trust the inner healer. This example doesn't show that Peter failed or was not a good candidate for psilocybin therapy. What it suggests to me is that he either didn't take a high enough dose of psilocybin—in my experience, those who get stuck in physical discomfort have not crossed the threshold of treatment—or that his inner healer was not ready for the work. We cannot push ourselves to heal deep-seated trauma; we must wait for the inner healer to reveal itself.

Creating Awareness

When you feel tightness in your body, nausea, or any other physical symptom when talking about emotions or trauma, that is your body talking to you. Learning how to listen is valuable. Perhaps you instantly shut down after someone says something that triggers you. Other times you might have a physical response. A counselor I once had asked me to close my eyes, put my hands on my heart, and breathe as she guided me in a self-love meditation. At the time the idea of bringing self-love to myself was so far-fetched that I began to hyperventilate. I was shocked at my response, and it took a while to wrap my head around it. But bringing your awareness around these physical and behavioral symptoms is the first step toward understanding them.

Finding the connection between how your body *feels* when you rub up against your shadow is an awareness that can be insightful. For me, I often feel a tightness in my throat and chest, and I notice my heart racing, when I'm crossing into shadow territory. My shadow tends to protect me through my voice. In the past that consisted of lashing out with hurtful words to push away whatever was threatening to make me feel too much of that all-too-familiar unconscious pain. Bringing awareness to the emotion-body connection can help us bring unconsciousness to consciousness.

The next time you notice an emotional trigger:

✦ Identify your surroundings. Where are you?

✦ Identify who you are interacting with. Is it this person or the situation? What was said or done that triggered you?

✦ Take 5 minutes, sit down, breathe, and contemplate the root of why this triggered you. What didn't you like about it? How did it make you feel? Did it remind you of anything, such as a past experience?

The more you take time to do this, the more your inner healer will grow.

Summary

The shadow is the part of the unconscious rejected by our ideal, otherwise known as our ego. Shadow work involves finding and bringing these unconscious thoughts, patterns, and behaviors to a conscious understanding for healing. Shadow work is the commitment to look deeply at the parts of ourselves we have rejected. It is the process of unpacking that backpack. It is the attempt to find meaning in and acceptance of these hidden parts so we can validate them and integrate them back into the whole where they belong. It's not easy work, and the path can be filled with obstacles.

Talk therapy is helpful when doing shadow work, but talk therapy alone can be a real struggle for those with hefty protectors in place. Psilocybin therapy, on the other hand, can break you wide open and often results in changes in one's life. This is why it is often said that one psychedelic session is like ten years of talk therapy. If balanced mental health is a struggle in your life, perhaps this type of therapy is worth considering.

CHAPTER 9

Microdosing

THE *NEW YORK TIMES, HARPER'S BAZAAR*, and *Huffington Post* are just a few of the large publications that have published pieces on microdosing as of late, and new books on the subject are being published regularly. Microdosing is the ingestion of very tiny doses of psychoactive substances that do not produce psychedelic effects. In this book I'm strictly speaking of psilocybin, but many other psychedelics have been used to microdose. As with most things psilocybin, microdosing is another aspect of treatment to examine closely and determine what may or may not be of benefit for you.

I first read about this practice in Ayelet Waldman's book, *A Really Good Day: How Microdosing Made a Mega Difference in My Mood, My Marriage, and My Life*, her memoir about microdosing LSD for a month. In the book, she talks about the demands of life and the emotional drawstrings of being a human, mother, wife, and professional. While all our stories are different, I quickly related to the feelings she shared. I have long struggled with melancholy and depression. Mixing these emotions into the demands of a professional career was one thing, but adding in the highs and lows of a long-term relationship and parenthood was another. Attempting to maintain sanity while trying to create a joyful life was hard. Some say modern parenting alongside modern life has led us to new extremes, which make it difficult to find balance or time to remember who we really are. We become guided by the roles we take on, as well as the ones society places upon us, and continue running on that hamster wheel until what . . . retirement? Death? We take endless photos so we don't miss anything, yet never pause long enough to capture a memory. I can't tell you how many times my children have relayed a memory of our lives that I don't recall. I attribute this to having a mind cluttered with so many thoughts and moving in so many directions at once that I simply don't acknowledge the need to record the memory.

When I discovered microdosing, I quickly recognized its ability to create space in my life. What I mean by that is that a tiny dosage of psilocybin can create what has been described as presence. This word, *presence*, has a lot of opportunities to trigger people. It's a word that has been thrown around in New Age circles for years, and if you've attended a yoga or meditation class you've probably heard it a lot. But I suggest you try to press pause on any feelings that might arise and consider the last time you truly felt present in your life. For me, it's extremely easy to list 100 reasons why I can't be present at any given moment: There's an email I need to reply to. I have patients to see. The house needs to be cleaned. The car needs an oil change. The roof just started leaking. An article I'm writing is due. I need to make dinner. I'm just so tired that I can't get off the couch. Being present is hard.

Although being busy and helping others fulfills me, the list of things to do gets longer and longer even though I've done a really good job at training myself to get the job done. This mind frame keeps me in a go-go-go state, cementing me into a role of productivity with the perceived image of a good parent, a responsible person, a dependable contributor, or whatever adjectives I can think of that drive my need to get everything done. This go-go-go state also steals away precious moments and memories from my life, making it harder and harder to connect and plug in to my life in meaningful ways.

I've found that microdosing is like pulling the stop lever to a large waterwheel. When you do it, all the water drains down as the wheel slows and eventually stops. You are no longer distracted by the water. In its place you see the incredible beauty of the constructed wheel. You can see it's made of the most beautiful wood and the craftsmanship is exquisite. You can watch the water glisten in its stillness. It is this perspective—this presence, this space—that I've seen microdosing create.

Microdosing seems to encourage us to look in new directions. It doesn't make us reject that list of things to do, but instead it relegates the list to its proper place—some things truly need to get done, and others aren't as imperative as we make them out to be. Once we have the space to recognize how often we fill our days with tasks rather than connection, we tend to start gravitating toward connection. The experience I'm trying to convey is a very subtle one and will vary from person to person.

Like changing a lens on a camera, microdosing enables us to take a step back and take stock of the big picture. We don't just see ourselves in a new way; it also alters how we think, feel, and react. Parents who microdose have reported the ability to recognize reactions in their children not as behavioral disruptions, but as their inability to express themselves. We often put very unrealistic expectations on our children to "use your words" or "just tell me how you are feeling." But let's be honest: how many of us had the mental or emotional capacity to verbalize complex human emotions at a young age? Few of us were even given the skills to learn how to do so, and we are not hardwired to know how. Through this new lens, parents have reported a greater opportunity for compassion and a truer sense of understanding their children when they may be struggling.

Every child—and every person, really—wants to be seen. I can't tell you how many times a day one of my kids asks me to "watch this, mom." When we are seen and actively listened to, we feel valued. The joy that microdosing can ignite provides a greater bandwidth to include moments of connection through play and interaction, as you are reminded of the fact that fun can be had in the simple passing moments of a day. Even if you don't have children, the simple ability to enjoy life is often ignited. When we take our foot off the gas a bit, we are reminded to loosen up. Microdosing reminds us of who we are and how we truly want to be in the world, subtly uncovering and releasing a version of ourselves that has grown bogged down over time. We all shift as we get older, but at times that shift is unintentional and almost blindingly subliminal. Whether we adopt grown-up roles and personas or curate ourselves to fit into society, we often take on layers that aren't a true reflection of who we are on the inside.

In a therapeutic setting, clinicians generally recommend microdosing to improve mental health, cognitive function, and academic and athletic performance, as well as to reduce stress and neurodegenerative diseases. There are two considerations with microdosing. First, those who are colorblind tend to get tracers with microdosing that can last for days afterward. There are also mixed results for those diagnosed with anxiety. Some have reported relief, while others have reported a worsening of their symptoms. And with anxiety it's often best to start with a very low dose.

Research has shown that psilocybin affects the 5-HT2A serotonin receptor, but does it do that in microdose amounts? It turns out it does. Doses as small as 0.1 to 0.5 grams of dried mushrooms have been reported to affect over half of the serotonin receptors at the neuronal synaptic sites. While a macrodose effects a larger percentage of serotonin receptors, it was surprising to learn that a microdose works at this level of efficiency.

Many sources mention that a microdose is one-tenth of a macrodose, but I find this confusing. As we've discussed, set and setting play a major part in the psilocybin experience, regardless of the dosage amount. As a naturopathic physician, I also know that standardizing a dose can be difficult because there will always be a percentage of the population who needs larger or smaller dosages. So instead of suggesting one-tenth of a macrodose as a standard—especially if you have no idea what your macrodose should be—my recommendation is to start at 0.3 grams of dried mushrooms and work your way up from there, as needed. Remember, dried mushrooms and synthetic psilocybin are not a straight gram to milligram conversion.

Microdosing will have no psychedelic effects because the amounts ingested are too small to shut down the default mode network in the brain. Hence no big epiphanies, hallucinations, or gigantic intrapersonal moments. But since serotonin is still being targeted—just in a

Ancestral Microdosing of Psilocybin

....

There is no reason to believe that psychedelic mushrooms weren't around in prehistoric times. It's quite possible that, through thousands of years of trial and error of taking these substances, our ancestors learned how to find relief from suffering and perhaps have periods of enlightenment through ceremony, passing this knowledge down through the generations.

In *A History of Medicine*, Plinio Prioreschi reviewed the traditional uses of psychedelics by Indigenous cultures. He mentioned the use of these substances in lower dosages for alleviating hunger, inspiring courage, reducing pain, and as an aphrodisiac.

Somehow, between then and now, perhaps due to misconceptions surrounding mushrooms' toxicity, we have forgotten this ingrained knowledge and how these low dosages could be beneficial in our daily lives. Thankfully, we are now regaining that knowledge.

smaller way—microdosing often results in a positive change in mood. Those who have been a part of clinical microdosing trials and those who have simply tried it on their own say that, overall, they just feel better: a little more pep to their step, more patience, a willingness to stop what they're doing to be present with another person. But if it were solely a serotonin response, this wouldn't explain the perceptions that seem to result from microdosing.

Psilocybin Microdosing Protocols

Currently, there are two major experts in the microdosing field, James Fadiman and Paul Stamets. Fadiman is considered the grandfather of microdosing. His educated, sensical, and often humorous view of the subject makes him a favorite in the community. With a Ph.D. in psychology from Stanford, his journey has led to a colorful career deeply rooted in connecting us with the natural world. While much of the initial microdosing research has been anecdotal, Fadiman has been collecting data for decades. He coined the term *citizen science*, which he used for his early days of collecting countless studies in microdosing. By providing a questionnaire to self-administered participants, Fadiman gathered an immense amount of introductory insight into the use and efficacy of psilocybin microdosing. Through his research, which he collected in a book called *The Psychedelic Explorer's Guide: Safe, Therapeutic, and Sacred Journeys*, he proved the correlations between microdosing and mental health improvement. In short, people felt better. What does that mean? If they were depressed, they felt less depressed. If they weren't doing well in school, after microdosing they were able to focus more in class and do better on their exams. Problem-solving skills increased within professional settings, removing long-standing obstacles. Even athletes reported achieving new goals they had set for themselves.

Through his citizen and clinical research, Fadiman developed a microdosing protocol. This approach became known as the Fadiman protocol, which he humbly now accepts. The protocol, which lasts thirty days, is to take a microdose one day, then take two days off, and then repeat. So if you took your first dose on a Monday, your next dose would be on Thursday, then again on Sunday, and so on. His research showed that the effects of the microdose often lingered throughout the following day, and therefore the need to microdose multiple days in a row wasn't necessary (and in his joking way, "wasteful").

The Fadiman Protocol

The Fadiman Protocol was designed to be used for four consecutive weeks. Fadiman's goal was to help people keenly distinguish microdosing days from non-microdosing days, as well as microdosing periods versus non-microdosing periods. You begin on day 1 with your first microdose, 0.5 grams of dried mushroom. The second day is what is called the transition day, the day that you will most likely still feel the effects of the microdose. The third day is back to baseline, or your normal day. Then the cycle begins again, repeating for four weeks. Best practice is to take the psilocybin before 10:00 a.m. on an empty stomach, as microdosing can have a mild stimulant effect. Feel free to eat normally afterward.

Fadiman Protocol

Day 1: first microdosing day

Day 2: transition day

Day 3: normal day

Day 4: second microdosing day

Duration: 4 weeks

Rest: 2 to 8 weeks

The Stamets Protocol

Herbalists have long known the benefits of medicinal mushrooms such as *Cordyceps*, maitake (*Grifola frondosa*), and lion's mane (*Hericium erinaceus*). World-renowned mycologist Paul Stamets combined this knowledge with psilocybin microdosing to produce what many believe to be a heightened microdosing therapy. His protocol is centered around improving cognitive function and neurogenesis—basically to help you think and feel good while also growing new brain cells. This protocol combines 0.1 to 0.5 grams whole-mushroom psilocybin with 50 to 200 mg lion's mane and 100 to 200 mg vitamin B_3. Because of the three layers of ingredients, the protocol became known as the Stamets Stack.

Vitamin B_3 (niacin) helps your body make energy from what you eat, and it is commonly known to lower cholesterol and perhaps ease arthritis. But Stamets's attention was focused on niacin's brain-boosting abilities. He likes the vitamin's capillary dilation effect, which allows substances to more easily move across the blood-brain barrier. (Niacin can produce a flushing initially that will diminish with regular use.)

Since the majority of neurogenesis occurs at nerve endpoints, using niacin helps potentially stimulate neurogenesis by carrying the lion's mane and psilocybin directly into the brain.

Although you cannot yet purchase a packaged Stamets Stack product, my guess is you will be able to in the relatively near future. For now, most people purchase each item individually and then take one after the other. Lion's mane comes in both tincture (liquid extract) and capsule forms, and niacin is widely available in capsule form. Again, best practice is to take the three components before 10:00 a.m. on an empty stomach. You may eat normally afterward.

Stamets Protocol
Days 1–4: stacking days
Days 5–7: transition days
Days 8–11: stacking days
Days 12–14: transition days
Duration: 4 weeks
Rest: 2 to 8 weeks

After trying both the Fadiman and Stamets protocols, I ended up with something completely different. My personal experience showed me that I don't need to microdose every day or even every week. What ended up working best for me was a microdosing schedule that was unique to me. But if you remember nothing else, remember this: when it comes to microdosing, *less is more*.

Create a Microdosing Record

Before you begin any microdosing protocol, I would like to suggest that you make a commitment to documenting your experience. By keeping track of my responses to each microdose, I was able to identify how long my moods stayed elevated, how my sleep was affected, and which days I was more productive. I also correlated my schedule around my menses, which created a positive shift in both physical and mental symptoms. This is why I stress the importance of journaling or keeping track as you microdose. If you really want to get curious about how microdosing is affecting you over time, writing it down helps. If you are someone who likes to journal, you can buy an inexpensive one to track your experience. Otherwise, create a simple document that you can easily fill in each day or download a sample one from my website. Do your best to write in it every day, including the days in between your microdoses. Include the following categories to help you keep track of what you are or are not experiencing:

Dosage:

Time of day:

Energy level:

Ability to focus:

Irritation level:

Productivity:

Sleep:

Motivation:

Mood:

Put a scale to each category, such as a scale of 1 to 5, with 1 being poor and 5 being great. Recording this information daily and being able to reflect back on it will provide you with a clear picture of how microdosing is working for you. It will also help guide you to the best protocol for your mind and circumstances.

Functional Mushrooms

Functional (or medicinal) mushrooms are not psychedelic. Instead, these mushrooms promote the health and vitality of our physical body. Paul Stamets's company, Fungi Perfecti, was one of the first to introduce functional mushrooms onto the wellness market. Maybe you've heard of reishi mushrooms (*Ganoderma lucidum*), but there are many medicinal mushrooms, including lion's mane, cordyceps, turkey tail (*Coriolis versicolor*), chaga (*Inonotus obliquus*), and maitake. The fruiting bodies of functional mushrooms have been used by many different cultures for thousands of years. For instance, in my Western herbalist training, I learned them as reishi, cordyceps, and turkey tail but in my Chinese medicine program they were lingzhi, dong chong xia cao, and yun zhi. In many different parts of the world, fresh and dried mushrooms can be found at the local apothecary. While the United States has been slow to use mushrooms medicinally, research is starting to catch up and prove what so many of us know.

A study performed by Israeli researcher Solomon P. Wasser indicated that medicinal mushrooms possess over 130 potential healing functions.[1] They are high in polysaccharides that show antitumor activity, and they contain beta-glucans that can prevent infection and support healing and chitin that activates the innate immune response. The antioxidant properties of functional mushrooms are mostly attributed to their ergothioneine properties and many make or help convert vitamin D, an important vitamin for gut and immunity health—not to mention mental health. Many functional mushrooms have been proven to reduce cholesterol through their natural statins, and some also include angiotensin-converting enzyme inhibitors. When we look at just this partial list, it is easy to classify mushrooms not only as medicinal but also as a superfood.

Lion's Mane

Lion's mane (*Hericium erinaceus*) is white and grows in long, thin strands that form a shaggy clump that somewhat resembles a lion's mane from the back. It is definitely distinct enough that when you see one, you'll be like, "Oh yeah! I see it."

Numerous studies have shown lion's mane's effectiveness in decreasing memory loss. Its two powerhouse compounds, hericenones and erinacines, have demonstrated the ability to protect the aging brain and help promote the creation of new neurons.

In my medical practice, lion's mane has been a particularly trusted ally for those with anxiety and mood swings, as backed up by research revealing its anti-inflammatory effects. My favorite study was one that had menopausal women eat cookies with lion's mane in them daily. Maybe it was just the cookies, but I think it was probably the lion's mane that lessened the subjects' anxiousness and irritation.

Cordyceps

There are nearly four hundred species of Cordyceps, some of which parasitize insects. *Cordyceps sinensis* is a powerful medicinal mushroom with a long history of use in traditional Chinese medicine. These light-to-bright-orange mushrooms resemble something akin to a sea coral with many outstretched tentacles slightly bending this way and that.

Cordyceps are well known in the naturopathic world for supporting cancer patients. One of the biggest benefits is their ability to lessen leukopenia, a drop in white blood cell count that leaves the patient susceptible to infection after chemotherapy. Cordyceps have shown the ability to stabilize white blood cell counts and help reduce fatigue.

Due to their antioxidant properties, cordyceps are often recommended to increase athletic stamina. They do this by increasing ATP—the body's form of energy—efficiently driving it to different parts of the body. The antioxidant effect has also been studied for its antiaging properties, with clinical research showing promise in both memory retention and increased physical strength.

Turkey Tail

Named because of its rounded, striped appearance, this mushroom's color ranges from brown to red. You can find turkey tail (*Coriolus versicolor*) in many North American forests, as it grows on most dead hardwood trees.

Turkey tail shines when it comes to supporting the immune system, which it does by increasing monocytes, a type of white blood cell that is particularly good at fighting infections. Turkey tail also stimulates macrophages—the cells in our body that eat up what shouldn't be there—making this functional mushroom another good choice for battling cancer.

A Chinese study also showed turkey tail's ability to reduce blood sugar levels and improve insulin resistance, making it a valuable consideration for treating type 2 diabetes.

Chaga

If you've ever walked through a forest of birch trees and seen a blackish-orange mass on a tree trunk, it may have been chaga (*Inonotus obliquus*). This spongy yet crumbly fungus doesn't look like a mushroom at all—it almost resembles a tumor on a tree.

Chaga has loads of antioxidants. Anecdotal evidence suggests that chaga can lower blood pressure and reduce inflammation in arthritis. It's antiaging properties are so beneficial you can now find chaga in many skincare lines. Lowering LDL (bad) cholesterol and raising HDL (good) cholesterol is another area that has drawn attention, and in Russia chaga is readily available in tincture form to treat cancer.

Caution is warranted, however. Chaga should be avoided if you are taking blood thinners, and it should not be taken within two weeks of having surgery. Also due to its high oxalate content, those who are prone to kidney and bladder stones should refrain from taking it.

Reishi

Reishi (*Ganoderma lucidum*) is a beautiful mushroom that looks as though it has been varnished to harden. The species is found in parts of the United States, Europe, and China, growing on decaying hardwood trees.

As one of the most popular of the functional mushrooms, reishi is also one of the most well researched. Studies have revealed reishi's beneficial anticancer properties and ability to reduce viral loads, treat thyroid disorders and hypertension, and provide liver support.

Reishi also serves as a sort of adaptogen, working to bring balance to the body and its functions. Whatever is low, reishi raises, and whatever is high, it lowers. Reishi works to modify the immune response: either calming it, should it be performing in an overly active state, or stimulating it if it is underperforming.

Maitake

In Japanese, maitake means "dancing mushroom." I love what Richard Dale Rogers says about maitake (*Grifola frondosa*) in his book *Medicinal Mushrooms: The Human Clinical Trials*: this name may be due to the appearance of the mushroom's shelved layers, or "humans joyfully leaping" when they find it growing at the base of trees. American mushroom foragers call it hen-of-the-woods, and it is typically found in the fall at the base of oak trees. Asian societies have included this fungus as part of their food cultures for thousands of years.

Maitake seems to have an affinity for balancing blood sugars and glucose in the body, making it a good candidate for adjunct diabetic therapy. With high beta-glucans present, it is another mushroom we consider when treating various cancers, and this is where human trials have been focused. Other research has seen higher rates of ovulation in patients diagnosed with polycystic ovary syndrome, decreased hypertension, and support in improving the liver's detoxification function.

Microdosing Functional Mushrooms

As an herbalist and naturopath, I've spent a lifetime mixing together different plants and mushrooms to create formulas. When curating a medicinal formula, there is an art to the blending. As with most things in life, you need to have a focal point for each formula—a foundation of purpose, so to speak. For example, if I was blending up a sleep formula, the focal point would be to induce sleep and therefore the main ingredients would include sleep-specific herbs or fungi. By including ingredients that nourish that focal point you also potentially treat the underlying cause of why you aren't sleeping well in the first place. Lastly, you need to mobilize all these ingredients by including herbs or fungi that stimulate them into action.

One thing I am learning about myself—and that I have often seen in my patients—is that less is more. Whether we are aware of it or not, our bodies can be quite sensitive and responsive to small doses of healing medicine. We actually don't need megadoses of natural substances to create positive and substantial shifts in our well-being.

My friend and fellow entrepreneur, Andrea Shuman, specializes in microdosing functional mushrooms. We were recently discussing this theory in conjunction with the art of blending mushrooms with herbs. Sometimes when you take a mushroom or medicinal herb alone, they don't always know which path you want them to follow in the body or which problem you want them to tackle. If we are taking gotu kola (*Centella asiatica*), for example, do we want it to provide clarity and focus to get through a busy day? Or are we looking for motivation to even get started? Maybe we are hoping it'll help heal the wound we got at last week's camping trip. My point is that without combining gotu kola with other herbs to "direct" it, so to speak, it can be hard to target and see obvious benefits.

While functional mushrooms have great healing potential, combining them with herbal medicine can provide clear direction for the medicine to reach our desired goal. Andrea says it best: "Microdosing function mushrooms singly is a lifeboat for many, but without an oar or a rudder. Without the tools to move you, you may end up adrift as you attempt to navigate treatment. Taking a microdose that is combined with helper herbs will act as the oar and rudder and help you safely ashore."

Let's look at the Stamets Stack as an example. The psilocybin would be the focal point, working to stabilize mood, increase energy, and promote clear thinking. The lion's mane is the nourisher. As a mushroom that works incredibly well to support our mental health and wellness, lion's mane nourishes the systems that contribute to these outcomes. And then you have niacin, which is most definitely the stimulator. Through its vasodilation, niacin drives the other two toward their actions.

Want to know more about microdosing functional mushrooms? Head over to my website, drjjpursell.com.

The Placebo Effect of Psilocybin

In October 2022, *Nature* magazine published an article that offered diminishing hope of microdosing efficacy. Although few full-scale microdosing trials have been conducted, the article portrayed a dismal portrait of its ineffectiveness. There is a lot to consider in this article, such as potentially poor design, inadequate dosing, isolation of active constituents, and duration. But it still leads us to question whether microdosing is effective or just a placebo. The placebo effect has long been a topic of conversation in medicine. If science cannot prove the validity of microdosing, it will forever be tainted as a reputable therapy. But as Fadiman can vouch, hundreds of thousands of people have reported positive changes in both their mental and physical health, such as diminished dysmenorrhea in women and migraine relief. Is that a "proof is in the pudding" example?

Summary

Science may never be able to corroborate citizen science's positive microdosing outcomes, but is that enough reason to put microdosing on the shelf? So many people are suffering from disconnection, debilitating anger, and depression. Microdosing psilocybin seems to find places where there is disequilibrium in the body and work to find equilibrium. As a practitioner committed to helping ease the suffering of others with the tenet of "Do no harm," I believe that microdosing has proven its worth and value as a therapy enough to be considered.

CHAPTER 10

Medical Considerations with Psilocybin

AS A PHYSICIAN I TOOK AN OATH at my graduation to do no harm. Naturopathic physicians go beyond that basic principle and lay out the following six tenets of patient care:

1. **First, Do No Harm (*Primum non nocere*):** Naturopathic physicians choose the most noninvasive and least toxic treatments necessary for each patient.

2. **The Healing Power of Nature (*Vis medicatrix naturae*):** Naturopathic doctors recognize the body's inherent ability to heal itself, as well as the healing powers of nature.

3. **Identify and Treat the Causes (*Tolle causam*):** Naturopathic doctors identify, address, and remove the underlying causes of disease.

4. **Doctor as Teacher (*Docere*):** Educating and supporting patients on personal health management is an important role for naturopathic doctors. They empower patients to take responsibility for their own health and acknowledge the therapeutic value inherent in the doctor-patient relationship.

5. **Treat the Whole Person (*Tolle totum*):** This is a holistic concept that recognizes the body as an integrated whole. Because

naturopathic doctors treat the patient, not the disease, we look at the entirety of a person's health.

6. **Prevention (*Praevenic*):** Naturopathic doctors promote a focus on overall health, wellness, and disease prevention.

When I reflect on these principles, I can easily see how psilocybin therapy can fit into our toolbox of therapies. The goal of any therapeutic practice should be founded first in the principle of doing no harm. In my opinion, one of the best ways to achieve this is through informed education. When we talk about psilocybin and the potential risks for participants, there are a few things that need to be discussed to ensure that it is a viable treatment option. While there are many messages and advertisements beginning to circulate regarding psilocybin—and they will only continue to multiply—being informed of potential risks is necessary.

Physical Risks

Taking psilocybin can increase your heart rate, blood pressure, and respiratory rate, physical responses that should be considered before agreeing to move forward with a session. Most clinical settings monitor these readings throughout the session. You may be thinking "How obtrusive!" But I've never noticed a participant being distracted or uncomfortable with these procedures during a session or had them report feeling so afterward.

Almost seventy years of psilocybin clinical research has yielded few reports of severe adverse physical effects. Very little of that research, however, has focused solely on physical reactions to psilocybin, such that I unfortunately have little to report at this time. Naturally, as we move into legal therapeutic use, we will have more substantial evidence of the true potential risks and contraindications.

Some researchers have speculated that psilocybin may cause heart damage with long-term (several times a week) high-dose usage. This refers to a standard research extreme dose, which would not typically be used in normal settings. But because psilocybin activates the serotonin 5-HT2B receptor, there may be need for concern, particularly for those with diagnosed heart disease. Although the serotonin 5-HT2A receptor is where we tend to notice psilocybin's effects, 5-HT2B is also affected. The 5-HT2B receptor is located throughout the body, but across the heart in particular. A study of serotonin receptors and heart disease suggests that the long-term activation of this receptor leads to the formation of valvular strands that can lead to valvular heart disease.[1] But again, this is with *extreme* use. In a therapeutic psilocybin model, you would not be taking these quantities, nor would you be taking it with such frequency. But since we do not have the research and data, it is best to be cautious.

Several studies have examined if psilocybin or the metabolized form, psilocin, has cardiotoxic potential. With the reporting of cardiac arrhythmias, cardiac arrest, contractile dysfunction, and myocardial infarction after ingestion of high doses (over 3.5 grams) of synthetic psilocybin, researchers have begun to investigate.

One psilocybin study used an electrocardiogram (ECG)—a machine that records the electrical signal from the heart—to check for arrhythmias, where the heart beats too slowly, too quickly, or irregularly; coronary heart disease, where the heart's blood supply is blocked or interrupted by a build-up of fatty substances; or heart attacks, where the supply of blood to the heart is suddenly blocked. Their findings showed that high doses of psilocybin resulted in a prolonged QT wave, which reflects the time it takes for the lower chambers (ventricles) of the heart to contract and relax.[2] They concluded that psilocin may disturb cardiac ion channels—the little doors that help regulate the electrical current of the heart. When the door is left open for longer than it should be, the whole rhythm gets out of whack. With excessive doses of psilocybin, this study showed that the doors stayed open longer than normal, but the standard clinical dose of 2 to 3 grams (dried mushroom) did not produce any ECG abnormalities.

Lastly, I will share the most widely reported case of potential cardio-toxicity of psilocybin. Mr. Burton was a man in his seventies, a person who was open to new experiences and self-growth. He connected with a facilitator and had a successful MDMA session. Next, he wanted to try a psilocybin session. Shortly after ingesting the psilocybin, Mr. Burton experienced cardiac arrest and died. The initial autopsy report listed cardiotoxicity as the cause of death, but it was later changed to preexisting heart disease. This story, however, is so muddled at this point that I am not sure anyone will ever know what truly happened. It's unknown if he knew he had a heart condition or if he was on medication. Perhaps the previous MDMA session triggered a cardiac response he was unaware of, but it also could have been purely coincidental timing.

Whatever the case may be, those with known heart conditions should consult with their cardiologist before embarking on a psilocybin session. As psilocybin medicine returns to the mainstream, my greatest concern is a lack of knowledge on the part of facilitators and a lack of education on the part of participants. My goal is to ensure that everyone who facilitates is fully educated on the potential risks and shares them with participants.

There are also reports of liver damage after eating *Psilocybe cubensis*, but the reports that I found mention "wild mushrooms" without proof of proper identification. Epilepsy is another controversial concern with regard to psilocybin use. After reviewing the literature, however, it seems that researchers are actually considering psilocybin as a therapeutic treatment for seizure disorders. Still, those with liver conditions or seizure disorders should consult their doctors before using psilocybin.

Potential Drug Interactions

The opioid painkiller Tramadol, cocaine, and amphetamines are all pharmaceuticals that are contradicted with psilocybin use. St. John's wort and yohimbe should be discontinued before using psilocybin as well.

What about antidepressants? There is a lot of discussion regarding this topic. I'll mainly focus on selective serotonin reuptake inhibitors (SSRIs) because they, like psilocybin, affect the serotonin receptors. Common SSRIs include citalopram (Celexa), escitalopram (Lexapro), fluoxetine (Prozac), fluvoxamine (Luvox), paroxetine (Paxil), and sertraline (Zoloft). Some antidepressants, like bupropion (Wellbutrin), do not affect serotonin.

Serotonin is released by neurons and then reabsorbed after a period of time. SSRIs basically block the reuptake channels so that serotonin gets to hang out longer. If serotonin is forced to hang out in the synaptic space longer, then more is ultimately available for the receiving receptor to suck up. Having more available to suck up increases mood, brain function, and clarity of thought.

SSRIs also offer a couple of bonuses. Depression and inflammation often go hand-in-hand, and research shows SSRIs also have anti-inflammatory effects. This physiological combination may be nature's way of trying to get us to slow down to rest, heal, and reset. Another advantage of SSRIs is their proven ability to increase neuroplasticity—the ability of neural networks in the brain to change through growth and reorganization. Psilocybin has this effect as well. Both classes of drugs are modulated by serotonin, and therefore both are able to help the brain form new neural pathways and adapt or respond differently to old experiences.

The big question is should you stop SSRIs before you partake in a psilocybin session? This is where I strongly advise medical consultation, because the answer is not cut and dry. Working with someone who is knowledgeable about both antidepressant medication and psilocybin work is best. In a study performed at the University of Basel, the researchers concluded that the inclusion of the SSRI Lexapro before a psilocybin session had no effect on the psilocybin effects measured.[3] But surprisingly what it did do was lessen commonly reported adverse psilocybin effects such as nausea, fatigue, anxiety, and headache. This study concluded that Lexapro and psilocybin can be safely administered together. Caution is still warranted, however, because this is only one study in a relatively new therapeutic space.

We must also consider that those who have been on SSRIs long-term have fewer receptor sites available. Unfortunately, a side effect of taking SSRIs over time is that the number of serotonin receptor sites diminishes. Because psilocybin drives up the amount serotonin to be sucked up, if you have fewer receptor sites to absorb it, you may have a diminished experience compared to someone who still has the normal number of receptors. Based on the scientific evidence, it has been proposed that chronic SSRI users may need a 30 to 50 percent higher dose than those not on a SSRI.[4] I often think of this principle when I hear of people who take an average psilocybin dose yet fail to experience anything.

One last thing regarding SSRIs: since early research is showing potential compatibility with psilocybin use, it may be relieving for those who need SSRIs to remain mentally stable before and after psilocybin therapy. To request that someone discontinue their SSRI treatment when it stabilizes their daily life is a risk that should not be taken lightly. Some doctors have suggested that remaining on an SSRI has the potential to create a balanced frame of mind from which one can be able to proceed safely into a psilocybin experience.

The last consideration is to remember that having the right frame of mind can make or break a session. It is not advisable to go into a session if there has been a recent upheaval in your life, such as the loss of a job, a breakup, or a death in your family. While psilocybin is regarded as a treatment for depression, if that depression is not stable it could weight a psilocybin session with challenges.

Serotonin Syndrome and Monoamine Oxidase Inhibitors

Serotonin toxicity—also known as serotonin syndrome—is a rare condition that occurs when there is too much serotonin in the body, and as a result your body goes into overdrive. All facilitators need to be on the lookout for symptoms, and participants need to be educated about this condition. One difficult thing is that mild and some moderate serotonin syndrome symptoms mimic psilocybin effects, such as nausea, diarrhea, headache, shivering, or increased heart rate and blood pressure. Mild cases will resolve, but moderate to severe cases should be treated immediately. Thankfully, there are typically no long-term or lasting complications of serotonin syndrome.

Although research shows a low risk for serotonin syndrome when psilocybin is used in combination with SSRIs, the use of monoamine

Symptoms of Severe Serotonin Syndrome

·················

High fever (above 102°F)

Seizure

Loss of consciousness

Muscle spasms/jerking

Lethargy

High blood pressure (above 140/90)

Irregular heartbeat

Severe confusion or disorientation

oxidase inhibitors (MAOIs) puts a participant in a higher risk category.[5] The most common MAOIs are isocarboxazid (Marplan), moclobemide (Manerix), phenelzine (Nardil), selegiline (Emsam), and tranylcypromine (Parnate). These drugs follow a different chemical pathway than the classic SSRIs and can actually increase responses to psilocybin. Those taking MAOIs should consult a medical professional before they consider using psilocybin.

Mental Health Contraindications

There is much discussion regarding mental and psychiatric diagnoses such as bipolar disorder and schizophrenia and the use of psilocybin. When I asked both Bill Richards and Michael Mithoefer why these groups have been excluded from clinical trials, they both reported it was because the FDA or clinical trial parameters excluded them. While that is a reasonable enough answer, it leaves a lot of room to ponder if psilocybin would help or hurt these populations.

David E. Gard and colleagues reviewed hundreds of case studies on the potential for the use of psilocybin, LSD, ayahuasca, and DMT to initiate a manic or psychotic episode.[6] They identified seventeen cases of such episodes that may have been related to a diagnosis of bipolar disorder or using the substance repeatedly in a relatively short period, suggesting the need for caution in those who suffer from bipolar disorder or have a family history of such.

Possible Long-Lasting Effects

For a very small percentage of participants, persistent psychosis and flashbacks might arise. These two symptoms often occur together and have been classified as hallucinogen-persisting perception disorder. The persistent psychosis, which I realize sounds terrifying, is a combination of disorganized thinking and paranoia. The inability to think clearly or return to the flow of one's life after a psilocybin session often leads to mood disturbances. In conjunction with these symptoms, someone might also have hallucinations or residual visual disturbances like halos or trails on moving objects. After much time reviewing the research and literature, I have found that less than 1 percent of the population that uses psilocybin will have a persistent psychosis outcome. After countless hours of searching, I was only able to find one person who had experienced persistent psychosis for a time after a psilocybin session. In this person's opinion, it was more of a reflection back on his poor set and setting and how it had taken him on the most unpleasant of journeys. As a result, he remained fearful for a period of time afterward.

A lack of integration sessions after a psilocybin session may also lead to what feels like depression, mental confusion, or an uncertainty of what to do with the things that arose during a session. Without the opportunity to talk about your experience, vital aspects of knowledge, learning, and growth can be missed, which can lead to feeling stuck or sad—mostly because a mountain of potential healing was unearthed but, without the proper processing, it simply remains in a pile. You still might be able to see it, but it is dense and compacted and all on top of itself.

If you'd like a concise checklist of all the above considerations, head over to my website for a free download.

Summary

As we move into this new landscape of therapeutic psilocybin, we have an abundance of historical use alongside a lot of avenues that remain to be explored scientifically. The biggest medical considerations before undergoing psilocybin therapy are cardiac disease and mental health diagnoses such as bipolar disorder and schizophrenia. Those on SSRIs should consult with a trained facilitator regarding options. Though psilocybin therapy may seem like untrod medical terrain, remember that psilocybin has been used for centuries. You don't have to look far to see the innate trust and relationship that countless cultures have with this magic mushroom. While we are in a modern age, facilitating in a modern way, recognizing and accepting the wisdom of the past and all those who used this medicine before us should carry significant value.

CHAPTER 11

Preparing for a Psilocybin Session

AS A NATUROPATHIC PHYSICIAN, I'm trained to think outside the box of Western medicine. While I diligently use my Western medicinal tools and skills, there is often so much more to consider. Entering a psychedelic session is no different. In this chapter I'll discuss important considerations to contemplate before and after a session, including nutrition, supplementation, and genetic issues.

Nutrient Deficiencies and How They Inhibit Biochemical Pathways

Fully understanding the chemistry of our bodies is an incredible advantage when approaching how to prepare for a psilocybin session, but it's a bit more than I have time for in this book. Instead I'll refer you to the work of the psychiatrist Dr. Julie Holland, who has authored books specifically on this subject, including *Good Chemistry: The Science of Connection, from Soul to Psychedelics*.

What I want to focus on is how nutrient deficiencies might affect how psilocybin processes in the body. Our bodies rely on a lot of different biochemical pathways to operate successfully—the metabolic pathway is one that you are probably familiar with. These pathways are like IKEA furniture instruction manuals, with one step leading to the next and so on. For each step to be a success, you need something: a screw, a bolt, or the next piece of whatever you're building. Without any of these components you cannot move on to the next step. In biochemical pathways, the screws and bolts are often vitamins and minerals that get added in at certain steps and allow the pathway to proceed.

Due to the paucity of nutrients in the world's food supply, even when eating organic and incorporating a healthy variety of foods, it remains difficult to supply your body with all the things it needs. Researchers have estimated that over 90 percent of the American population has nutritional deficiencies, noting that most common medical conditions are due to this problem. Testing is one challenging part of diagnosing these deficiencies, as many regular blood tests will not show overt, or pathological, results. Understanding the difference between deficiency, insufficiency, and sufficiency is important. Having enough of a nutrient to survive is very different then having enough to fuel all the parts of the system and is even farther from having enough to thrive. Let's look at an example. A typical lab test gives the reference range for vitamin B_{12} as 190 to 950 picograms per milliliter, which is quite a wide range. If you get a blood test and your B_{12} level is 200 picograms per milliliter, it will read as normal, and no intervention will typically be offered. As a naturopath, I look at that level and read it as insufficient. Yes, you have some, but the probability that you have enough to run biochemical pathways is low. (If you'd like to know more about nutrient deficiencies or want to be tested by a reputable company, check out my website.)

Everything runs through a biochemical pathway, including psilocybin. Vitamin C, vitamin B_6, amino acids, and folate are just a few of the minerals, vitamins, and nutrients needed for our bodily systems to be able to function at their best, including when we are processing psilocybin. When we are deficient in any of these nutrients, certain pathways begin to get derailed or inhibited all together. In the case of preparing for a psilocybin session, we want to support our metabolic and detoxification pathways beforehand. Ensuring that you have sufficient cofactors—the pieces, screws, and bolts—will not only keep the process moving along but will support the natural detoxification of your body afterward.

Epigenetics and Genetic Factors

Epigenetics is the study of how our behaviors and the environment cause changes to our DNA that affect the way our genes function—whether they are turned on or turned off. How our bodies adapt to modern life also affects our genes. For example, the lack of nutrients in the food we eat affects our biochemical pathways. When insufficiencies or outright deficiencies go on for long periods of time, a gene may turn on or off in an attempt to adapt. Recent studies have shown that epigenetics plays a central role in many types of diseases, including cardiovascular diseases, neurological diseases, metabolic disorders, and cancer. Naturally keeping up with our health is the best way to prevent epigenetic change.

Another genetic factor to consider with regard to the use of psychedelics is the single nucleotide polymorphism (SNP), which represent a mutation in a single nucleotide, a DNA building block. As Ben Lynch says, "I consider SNPs the 'spice of life.' They contribute positively to genetic variation and allow us to act differently, experience things differently, and adapt differently." SNPs are very common—each of us has about 50,000 of them. Although most of these mutations do not matter, there are times when they do.

Knowing our genetic code can provide insight into our mental and physical health. By utilizing the raw data of ancestry tests such as 23andMe, software programs can let us know which considerations to make in our health plans. We can even utilize this science to get specific about nutrients and if there is a reduced (or increased) ability for a vitamin, mineral, or other cofactor to bind. For example, I recently had a patient with an SNP in the gene responsible for choline production. Long-term choline deficiency can lead to muscle and liver damage, as well as fatty deposits in the liver. Short-term insufficiency/deficiency can lead to generalized fatigue, muscle aches, and memory decline, all of which she was experiencing. When we utilize modern tools of medicine, we can curate health care like never before.

In the case of genomics and psychedelics, there are several mutations that should be considered, but I'll refer to three that have been researched as of late. The first is one named CYP450, a cytochrome enzyme found in the liver and gut. A mutation in this gene can affect how we process psilocybin. Catechol-O-methyltransferase is an enzyme involved in the metabolism of neurotransmitters like dopamine, epinephrine, and norepinephrine. SNPs in the gene coding this enzyme have been well studied, and a deficiency in the enzyme has been correlated to a decrease in psychedelic metabolism. Another mutation to examine is in the serotonin 5-HT2AR gene, which can also influence how psilocybin is processed. One study examined seven SNPs in relation to this gene.[1] They concluded that these SNPs produced statistically significant, although modest, effects on the efficacy and potency of psilocybin, LSD, mescaline, and 5-MeO-DMT. This early research shows the value of genomics in relation to psychedelic therapy. I'm sure the research in this field will grow so that we may better understand participant's varying experiences with standardized dosages.

If you have the means to get a comprehensive genetic test completed, I recommend it. It isn't necessary before a psilocybin session but it can provide insight into neurotransmitter and detoxification function. Once again, my website provides resources for trusted genetic testing companies.

One Month Before a Session

Here is a sample protocol of supplements to be considered during the month before a psilocybin session. These supplements are meant to be supportive and nurturing to the body in preparation for therapy. Before initiating a supplement regimen, please consult with your health care professional to ensure the supplements are safe for your health profile.

N-acetyl cysteine (500 mg per day) is used by many people before a session to increase glutathione, which protects both the gut and brain from oxidative stress.

Acetyl-l-carnitine or Na-R-ALA (250 to 500 mg per day) are amino acids that help reduce free radicals, support mitochondria, and increase GABA and glutamate absorption (which are calming and reduce inflammation) from psilocybin.[2]

A bioavailable form of magnesium such as citrate or glycinate (200 to 400 mg per day) can be very helpful to reduce certain symptoms, such as tension in the body and jaw, and can reduce the potential for increased heart rate during a session. If this dosage results in loose stools that don't resolve after three days, cut the dose in half.

Vitamin C (1000 mg per day) is a great supplement to protect the liver from toxicity. To some degree, psilocybin is a natural toxin, and the liver is responsible for filtering that out afterwards. Vitamin C helps with that process.

Vitamin B_{12} is an important cofactor for methylation. Methylation is an important biochemical process in the body which supports the nervous, cardiac, and immune systems, as well as detoxification. Ensuring your methylation pathways are running strong beforehand improves immunity and supports detoxification afterwards. I typically recommend a B complex that includes B_6 and folate in a liquid form. Dosage varies depending on the product.

Oral lavender (100 mg of a supplement containing 25 to 46 percent linalool) is a good supplement for calming anxiety in the weeks leading up to the session.

Two Weeks Before a Session

About two weeks before a session, start preparing your mind for session day. If you are up to it, use a journal and write down your thoughts for later reflection. Extracting the thoughts from our heads and getting them onto a page can be very beneficial. Allow time and space to contemplate the journey ahead.

It's also important to get your body prepared. During the two weeks before a session, get plenty of sleep, be mindful of your water and food intake, and consider taking herbal supplements to promote healthy liver function, ward off illness, and combat any nervousness you may be experiencing.

Rest

It goes without saying that proper sleep is vital for a healthy body. Not only does it help us have the energy to get through the day, but sleep is when our body detoxifies. This precious time is when the liver goes to work processing out what isn't needed and building up what we need for the next day. Try to get eight hours of sleep a night.

Hydration

When you are properly hydrated, the water in your body helps deliver nutrients to your cells, aids in organ function, and supports the regulation of body temperature. It is vital to support these physiological processes when taking psychedelics. You should be consuming, at a minimum, half of your body weight in ounces each day. For example, if you weigh 120 pounds, you should be consuming 60 ounces of water daily.

Diet

Filling your diet with foods that fuel and support your body's functioning can make a marked difference in how you feel after a psychedelic session. Eating a rainbow of fruits and vegetables of various colors and rich in antioxidants will help you feel supercharged. In addition, daily fiber intake supports both cellular health and proper elimination, so shoot for an average of 30 grams every day.

In general, lowering your overall bodily inflammation will aid the process of any medical procedure, whether it's surgery, routine exams, or a psychedelic session. When inflammation is high, the body's energy is pulled in a lot of different directions to lower it. If inflammation is leading to physical pain, further energy is recruited, taking it away from other bodily functions. Stabilizing your body before taking psychedelics helps the process, both during and after the session.

Eating a balanced diet and making dietary choices that are low-inflammatory will lower the body's overall inflammation. This includes healthy proteins, fresh produce, and foods such as nuts and fish that are rich in omega-3 and omega-9 fatty acids. Avoiding processed sugars and saturated fats also aids this process. When your inflammation is lower and you take a psychedelic substance, the body has a better ability to be focused on that process.

The Liver and Elimination Pathways

Any substance we consume is broken down into things our body keeps and waste it shuttles out. The liver—the master detoxifier of the body—is the human body's primary filtration system. It identifies toxins in the blood and breaks them down into waste. The liver also releases an enzyme, known as alkaline phosphatase, which plays a role in psilocybin-to-psilocin conversion. Ensuring the liver and elimination pathways are functioning well will improve how you feel both during and after a session. Nightly castor oil packs are an easy way to support the liver. This topical application is easy to do, as well as inexpensive. There is a step-by-step how-to guide on my website. If you'd like to learn more ways to support the liver and elimination pathways, check out my first book, *The Herbal Apothecary: 100 Medicinal Herbs and How to Use Them*. It is loaded with great information about these systems, specific herbs to support them, and recipes you can make at home.

Regarding what to avoid, we know St. John's Wort speeds up hepatic metabolism and grapefruit slows it down, so consider eliminating both of these during the two weeks prior to a session.

Stay Well

Getting sick right before a planned session is always a bummer. To keep your immune system active and prevent illness, I recommend using an herbal or functional mushroom supplement to ward the ick away. Consider using herbs like ashwagandha, elder, boneset, thyme, and rosemary in a tea, tincture, or supplement form. There are also preblended mixtures out there for immune support. The same goes for functional mushroom supplements: reishi, lion's mane, and chaga are all good choices to use before a session.

Nervousness

To combat any nervousness you may be feeling, try drinking chamomile tea in the evening for two weeks beforehand. Alternatively, you might take an herbal supplement with oats, passionflower, catnip, lemon balm, or skullcap. These nervines are safe to consume before a session and will help to relax the nervous system, which often calms anxiety or nervousness.

During a Session

Typically I'll work to help the participant get through a nausea wave, and I like to have ginger tea or chews available if the participant feels inclined.

After a Session

The night after a session, have some electrolytes on hand to hydrate. For two to seven days afterward, consider taking L-tyrosine (500 mg twice daily). While psilocybin appears to focus on serotonin receptors, PET scans suggest a secondary effect—an increase in brain dopamine concentrations. After a session, this could lead to a dramatic drop in dopamine. Taking exogenous L-tyrosine supports amino acid production of natural dopamine to maintain proper neurotransmitter levels.

Summary

When the time comes, most of you could easily enter a psilocybin session without all this preparation. But I do think it is wise to support your body both physically and mentally beforehand. Perhaps you'll even adopt some of these healthy lifestyle suggestions long-term. Many believe health must be an all-in commitment, commitment to body, mind, and spirit. And there are times in our lives that require that level of commitment. But I believe, if we are generally in good health, the idea is to do the best we can. Make healthy choices for yourself as often as you can. It truly is all about balance. As always, please contact me if you have any questions, as I'm happy to clarify or explain further.

CHAPTER 12

Respect and Ethics

I HAVE SEVERAL PLACES IN MY HOME that I write from—I've never been a "one desk" type of woman, much preferring to move from spot to spot, depending on my mood. Today I am in the sunroom. I sit in a slightly oversized chair that used to be my mom's, and the indirect light is coming in from all sides of me. I have many houseplants in this area, including a few that I've nearly killed due to improper care and then desperately fought to bring back from the brink of death. My chair has a good vantage over the rest of the house, which means I can see if my kids try to sneak into the kitchen for snacks they aren't supposed to have or if my dog wants to go outside. It is a good place to think, in this seat. And when I think about topics such as psychedelic ethics and integration, my thoughts can go on for hours. I definitely don't have all the answers, and some of my thoughts are bound to shift and change as I continue down this path. My goal is to ignite important conversations. In my exploration of the following topics, all I can do is be open and vulnerable and share my personal thoughts on these vitally important issues.

Ethics is such a modern word when we think about it. While many of our scholarly ancestors such as Aristotle and Plato discussed the topics of "living well" or "living right," they used different Greek words to describe what is now known as *ethical*.

Since I have no cultural ties with the ways in which the ancestors and originators of psilocybin medicine ethically held the medicine, I can only draw from my studies and experiences in the modern-day community. As part of a community, you are most assuredly held to account for the ways in which you live. If you live within the ways of "living well," you are in union with the greater community and their needs and goals. Should you stray from the values of the community in a way that causes harm or creates separation, there is an established order to handle the transgression. In Europe and North America, we established laws, regulations, licenses, and about every type of bureaucracy you could imagine. And despite this, there are a lot of people who continue to stray from "living well."

Facilitator and Participant Ethics in Psychedelic Therapy

As psychedelic medicine returns to the mainstream Western medicine model, there will be a huge need for facilitators and practitioners to guide sessions. We've already seen growing psychedelic tourism—and the psychedelic harm that has resulted from some of these enterprises. While there is a strong push to reschedule psychedelic substances for medicinal purposes, our country is way behind in developing the foundation that will be needed to actually use them. Training facilitators is just one piece of that foundation. Another is a plan to protect both the participants and the facilitators.

As graduate students in the Certificate in Psychedelic Training and Research at the California Institute of Integral Studies, we talk about ethics a lot. How can we be leaders in an emerging field and ensure that all facilitators are trained and holding their clients in the safest ways of service? Who can participants go to should a facilitator fail to comply with safety measures or if questionable actions occurred during a session? If facilitators are working alone in private practice, who holds them accountable? And the inverse, where can facilitators go if they feel a participant displayed questionable behavior or put them at risk during a session? We currently don't have answers to these questions.

As of now, there is no regulating body for psychedelic medicine. I'm mentioning this not because it is a top priority to establish one.

Groups Supporting Ethics in the Psychedelic Space

·················

These professional organizations focus on upholding ethical practices in the psychedelic space:

+ American Association of Psychedelics (aapsychedelics.org)

+ American Psychedelic Practitioners Association (appa-us.org)

+ Board of Psychedelic Medicine and Therapies (psychedelicsboard.org)

+ Psychedelic Medicine Association (psychedelicmedicineassociation.org)

(I'm actually on the fence about more regulation.) But it will be up to participants to do their homework to find the right facilitator to ensure safety and competency. Do we need a certification board? Does passing an exam mean you are fully competent to help others in this space? If we look at the history, while passing an exam demonstrates intellect, it doesn't prove moral values. Do we need an ethical board to manage and investigate complaints? In Oregon, you currently only need a high school diploma and a certificate from a certified psychedelic training center to be a facilitator. How do we go about structuring the management process of complaints and the hierarchy of discipline within the profession? Do we require all facilitators to hold a professional degree of some sort and put their licensing board in charge of psychedelic matters within each profession? And if we do that, what about the amazing sitters, tribes, and religious leaders and communities who don't fit into this prescribed box we may be creating? I don't have the answers here, but I encourage you to pay attention and get involved should you find passion in this area. In the long run, there will be systems put in place—this is America, after all—and I think it is best that the right people (meaning a diverse and inclusive population) help establish whatever is on the horizon for the ethics of psychedelic medicine.

Ethics Board

At present, we have no ethics board that oversees the rising number of psychedelic medicine facilitators. Do we need one? Again, I ride the fence on this. As someone who has breathed and lived herbal medicine for over thirty years, I was there when herbal medicine went from unregulated to FDA-regulated. I understand the basic premise—let's protect people from harm. But in that policy change, many of us lost the right to make our own medicine and legally share it through commerce. This led to having to choose a side: either go bankrupt in attempting to get on the FDA bandwagon or fly under the radar to continue safely providing for our communities. I feel the same will happen with psychedelics and facilitators. Those who have sat as facilitators for years will continue to provide safely for their communities, while others will feel compelled to go the legalized facilitator route. But this divided profession will be nearly impossible to regulate, particularly from an ethical perspective. Perhaps this is why some psychedelic practitioners are persuading the current medical model to shift. Through regulated practices and environments, there are controls in place to minimize error. If we have standards for facilities, regulations around dosing, and state- or federal-approved training facilities, do we minimize the potential for human harm? I'm not sure we do. This is a topic of debate within the community, and I've no doubt it will continue to be for years to come.

As it stands now, facilitators who are board-certified (NDs, MDs, nurses, DOs, therapists, and such) will report to their licensing board for psychedelic malpractice and ethical complaints. But who will oversee unlicensed facilitators? MAPS has a code of ethics and an ethical review board for their research and training programs. Also recently formed is the Board of Psychedelic Medicine and Therapies, which is proposing a national certification test to be a registered facilitator. Oregon is proposing a state exam through a state-certified training course, but if your state hasn't legalized psychedelic therapy, I'm not sure what such a test would mean for you.

When a new therapy enters the Western medical model, we witness this process unfolding in real time, creating a lot of questions around how to proceed. The Oregon Psilocybin Advisory Board went through all of this, and as a witness I can say it was neither easy nor always unanimous. When we think about psychedelic substances and the healing they offer, we cannot just think of ourselves and how we judge it best to proceed. It takes an extremely competent person to view the task from multiple angles and be willing to consider what is in the best interest for all. A lot of the regulatory steps that are being set forth seem to be following a structure that, in my opinion, is outdated and founded in old ways of thinking that exclude marginalized peoples and religious leaders accustomed to psychedelic substance use. If we keep repeating the same bureaucracy in this modern world, the room for profound, healthy, and beneficial shifts that include everyone will be lost.

Psychedelics teach us there is more out there. More connection, more love, and more opportunities to bring new ideas to the table. Because of this, I struggle with putting psychedelic therapy in the same box as other medical models with regard to regulation and certification. Naturally, I want everyone to be safe while using these substances, but I also want to ensure everyone has access to them in a way that empowers.

Summary

Please choose your partner in psychedelic journeying wisely. Don't rush to the next retreat center advertised or assume that all facilitators are the same. Get involved in the psychedelic movement by paying attention to what is happening in your communities. Always respect the lineage holders of this medicine. Take time and find the right facilitator who can understand who you are and your background. Ultimately this is a relationship, one in which there is a huge opportunity to open up the healing process by being vulnerable and to let someone see all of the sides of who you are. While the idea of that might take your breath away and bring fear to your heart, the facilitator who walks the right path is eager and waiting to embrace you for *you*. So come as you are.

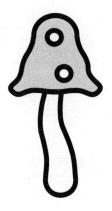

Other Psychedelics

As we continue down the path of the psychedelic medical model, there are other substances that are or will soon be added to the legalized system. Speaking with a certified health care professional about these substances is best, but I would like to introduce them here to provide some background.

Ayahuasca

- A hallucinogenic
- Illegal in the United States, except as part of sanctioned religious ceremonies
- Combination of two South American plants, typically caapi (*Banisteriopsis caapi*) and chacruna (*Psychotria viridis*)
- Generally drunk as a tea
- Common reports are connection with self, spirit, and others and deep psychological insights
- Duration range is 4–6 hours
- Most often used for treating depression and suicidal ideation, as well as achieving enlightenment, purpose, and connection
- Contraindications include bipolar disorder, psychotic disorder, and use with SSRIs, SNRIs, SPARIs, TCAs, trazodone (>150 mg), methadone, tramadol, lithium, and stimulants and neurotransmitter-releasing agents such as amphetamine, cocaine, MDMA, and cathinones

DMT (N, N-Dimethyltryptamine)

- A hallucinogenic and psychedelic
- Illegal in the United States

- A white crystalline powder derived from certain plants found in Mexico, South America, and parts of Asia, such as chacruna (*Psychotria viridis*); also synthetically manufactured
- Can be vaporized, insufflated, or injected
- Intense psychedelic and hallucinogenic experience
- Duration only 10 minutes
- Most often used for neurogenesis, depression, anxiety, and self-enlightenment
- Contraindications include advanced cardiovascular conditions, uncontrolled hypertension, and bipolar or psychotic disorders

5-MeO-DMT (5-Methoxy-N,N-Dimethyltryptamine)
- A psychedelic
- Illegal in the United States
- Sourced from parotid secretions of the Sonoran Desert (Colorado River) toad, *Incilius alvarius*. It can also be made synthetically.
- Generally crystallized, vaporized, or smoked
- Very powerful, can often feel as if merging with the infinite, eternal love, ego dissolution
- Duration about 15 minutes
- Most often used for anxiety and depression
- Contraindications include use of MAOIs, advanced cardiovascular conditions, uncontrolled hypertension, pregnancy, schizophrenia or bipolar disorder, and epilepsy or seizure disorder

Ibogaine
- A psychedelic with dissociative properties
- Illegal in the United States
- Extracted from the African iboga plant (*Tabernanthe iboga*) or synthetically manufactured
- Typically taken as a powder that is encapsulated, though some religions use the pulverized root
- Strong psychedelic with extremely intense experiences

- Duration is up to 24 hours
- Most often used for addiction to opioids, cocaine, or heroin
- Contraindications are extensive, including cardiac pathologies, methadone use, electrolyte issues, stimulant history, liver disease, epilepsy, pregnancy, brain pathologies, lung conditions, mental health diagnoses such as bipolar disorder and schizophrenia

Ketamine

- A psychoactive compound initially used as a dissociative anesthetic
- Currently legal in the United States
- Synthetically manufactured
- Several modes of administration, including intravenously, intramuscularly, intranasally, and orally
- Depending on dosage, session can be highly dissociative or at a lower dose used in conjunction with talk therapy
- Duration depends on mode of administration, but usually 15–30 minutes after onset
- Most often used for depression, addiction, and reduction of suicidal ideation
- Contraindications include cardiac pathologies, hypertension, and schizophrenia

LSD (Lysergic Acid Diethylamide)

- A psychedelic
- Illegal in the United States
- A synthetic powder that is then diluted into liquid
- Taken as a liquid or pressed into blotter paper (tabs)
- Stimulates euphoria and often accompanied by visual alterations
- Duration is typically 8–10 hours
- Most often used for depression, addiction, and achieving spiritual connection
- Contraindications include cardiac pathologies, hypertension, schizophrenia, and bipolar disorder

MDMA (Ecstasy, Molly)

- A psychedelic
- Currently illegal in the United States, but undergoing clinical trials
- Synthetically manufactured
- Generally taken in capsule form or intranasally
- Produces powerful feelings of empathy and compassion
- Duration is typically 3–6 hours, depending on dosage

Psilocybin Retreats and Costs

Since we have no long-term data on psilocybin session costs, what I share here is a glimpse into an ever-changing entrepreneurial terrain. Until recently, the only way to experience a psychedelic session was to either find an underground sitter or to travel to another country for a healing retreat.

Disclaimer: Neither I as the author or Timber Press as the publisher are affiliated with any of the following retreat centers and therefore cannot recommend one. The following list is strictly for information purposes.

Retreats are offered in individual settings as well as for couples and groups. The setting is typically an aesthetically pleasing environment curated to encourage the participant(s) to feel relaxed and safe. Costs for such experiences are typically in the $3000 to $10,000 range, depending on the services offered and the duration of your stay.

Oregon is now accepting applications for both facilitator and facilitation center licenses. Most of these will lead to private client services with a one-day experience model. This means you'll arrive in the morning, have your session, and return home afterward. Based on the little research I have, licensed professionals will likely charge somewhere in the $800 to $3500 range, with an average between $1000 and $3000. This fee should, at the minimum, include pre-session, session, and post-session check-in and integration.

While Oregon and other states are gearing up, here is a list of international retreat centers currently accepting participants for services.

Behold Retreats
- Based in Portugal and Costa Rica
- Retreat costs start at $5250

- Duration is 6 nights
- Behold specializes in intimate and highly curated psilocybin sessions and focuses on connecting participants to themselves and their higher purpose.

Buena Vida

- Based in Mexico
- Retreat costs start at $3350
- Duration is 7 days
- Buena Vida strongly believes in the spiritual lineage of psilocybin use and weaves it alongside modern use techniques. They also have a nice eight-week integration follow-up offered after the retreat.

Essence Institute

- Based in the Netherlands
- Retreat costs start at $1400
- Duration is 3 days
- This is a great option for a shorter retreat with a lower price tag. Homed in a beautiful area with forests and gardens, Essence utilizes psilocybin in combination with traditional therapies including breathwork, bodywork, yoga, mindfulness, meditation, and systemic work.

MycoMeditations

- Based in Jamaica
- Retreat costs start at $4300
- Duration is 7 nights
- MycoMeditations is known for its luxury accommodations and bridging the gap between traditional usage and modern applications. The staff has adopted research from Johns Hopkins University and Imperial College London to ensure a safe and effective transformative experience.

Zion Life Retreat

- Based in Jamaica
- Retreat costs are $2800 or $600
- Durations are 4 days or 1 day
- Guided by Stephanie Barnwell, an indigenous Gullah Geechee native from the Sea Islands in Beaufort. Stephanie is a nurse with more than twenty years of experience in guiding participants in psilocybin sessions.

Psychedelic Music Playlists

Music can make or break a psilocybin session. These tried-and-true playlists are a great place to begin your musical education regarding psilocybin sessions. Remember, a playlist that is well-thought-out gently leads the participant, like a guide, as the experience grows, peaks, and descends, ideally toward a beneficial outcome. The playlists I recommend are available on Spotify and are listed below by search name and playlist title.

Chacruna 2
- A Playlist for Psilocybin

Imperial College London
- Psychedelic Therapy Playlist 1
- Psychedelic Therapy Playlist 3

John Hopkins
- Music for Psychedelic Therapy
- John Hopkins Psilocybin Study
- John Hopkins Psilocybin Playlist

MAPS
- MAPS Playlist A
- MDMA Therapy Playlist

NYU
- Psilocybin Trial Playlist
- Session: Opening
- Session: Active

Psychedelic Harm Support

These groups are great resources to utilize to better understand psychedelic harm and to reach out to for support if you feel you have been a victim of poor practices.

Bluelight

bluelight.org/xf

DanceSafe

dancesafe.org

The Fireside Project

firesideproject.org

PsiloHealth

psilohealth.co

Psychedelic Survivors

psychedelic-survivors.com

Psygaia

howtousepsychedelics.com

TripSit

tripsit.me

The Zendo Project

zendoproject.org/resources

How to Become a Facilitator

By far, the most common question I get is "How can I become a psychedelic facilitator?" Here is a simple checklist to provide you with some direction. Because Oregon is the only state currently offering legalized psilocybin facilitation, I'll describe its guidelines.

To become a licensed facilitator in Oregon, you must:

+ be twenty-one years of age or older;

+ have a high school diploma or equivalent;

+ be an Oregon resident (this requirement expires in 2025);

+ pass a criminal background check;

+ complete a psilocybin facilitator training program with a curriculum approved by Oregon Psilocybin Services prior to applying for licensure; and

+ pass an exam administered by Oregon Psilocybin Services.

If you meet the basic requirements, the next step is to consider which program is right for you. As listed in the following section, there are plenty of programs available to choose from. Some programs have degree completion requirements, while others do not. Look into the programs and carefully consider their requirements and costs. I would also recommend getting some therapy training (such as cognitive behavioral or internal family systems therapy), which can be valuable in the integration process.

Once you complete a program, consider your options for moving your career forward. If you'd like to strike out as an independent facilitator, then you'll need to apply for a facilitation center license. Or perhaps you'd rather have someone else do all the paperwork and simply join an already established center. Which states are close to offering legal psilocybin therapy? Take all these things into consideration.

If you have further questions or want to talk through the process, don't hesitate to reach out to me.

Psychedelic Therapy Training Programs

Please note that this list will quickly become outdated as the profession grows, but it will continue to be a good reference of who was on the ground floor in the development of training curriculums for the therapeutic use of psychedelics.

Programs Outside of Oregon

California Institute of Integral Studies
ciis.edu
Established: 2015
Duration: 1 year
Format: online and in-person
Location: San Francisco or Boston
Cost: $9300
Advantages: MAPS MDMA training is folded into the curriculum, and leaders in the field teach courses

Fluence
fluencetraining.com
Established: 2019
Duration: varies
Format: online and in-person
Location: retreats are in New York state.
Cost: varies
Advantages: several options available to put together a focused area of study

Naropa University
naropa.edu
Established: 2021 (school was established in 1974)
Duration: 10 months
Format: online and in-person
Location: Boulder, Colorado
Cost: $10,000
Advantages: MAPS MDMA training is folded into the curriculum

Psychedelic Therapy Training
ubiquityuniversity.org/courses/phd-in-psychedelic-studies
Established: 2020
Duration: 3 years
Format: online and in-person
Location: global travel
Cost: approximately $50,000
Advantages: direct entry into traditional cultures with experiential training, master's and Ph.D. options

The Center for Psychedelic Psychotherapy and Trauma Research

icahn.mssm.edu/research/ center-psychedelic-psychotherapy- trauma-research
Established: 2020
Duration: retreats and short-term trainings available
Format: in-person
Location: New York City
Cost: varies
Advantages: in-person experience

The Psychedelic Sitters School

psychedelicsittersschool.org
Established: 2012
Duration: 4–6 months
Format: online and in-person
Location: Boulder, Colorado
Cost: $3950 to $5850
Advantages: experienced staff and trainers

....

Oregon-Approved Facilitator Training

Alma Institute

almatraining.org
Established: 2022
Duration: 6 months
Format: online
Location: Portland, OR
Cost: $11,750
Advantages: focus on indigenous history and use

Awaken ABA Psilocybin Facilitator Training

awakenaba.com
Established: 2022
Duration: 2 months
Format: online and practicum hours
Location: Oregon
Cost: $4500
Advantages: cost-effective

Changa Institute

changainstitute.com
Established: 2016, licensed in Oregon in 2022
Duration: 3 or 6 months (120 hours of curriculum)
Format: online and in-person
Location: Portland, Oregon
Cost: $9550
Advantages: aligned with the North Star Ethics Pledge, executive network community and immersive training to build confidence

Earth Medicine Center Training Program

earthmedicinecenter.com
Established: 2022
Duration: 12 months
Format: online and in-person
Location: Oregon
Cost: varies
Advantages: extensive curriculum

InnerTrek

innertrek.org
Established: 2022
Duration: 6 months
Format: online and in-person
Location: Portland, Oregon
Cost: $8500

SoundMind Institute

soundmind.training/program
Established: 2022
Duration: 12 months
Format: online
Location: Oregon
Cost: $11,300
Advantages: curriculum is physician designed and directed

Subtle Winds

subtlewinds.com
Established: 2022
Duration: 3 months
Format: online and in-person
Location: Eugene, Oregon
Cost: $9000
Advantages: solid curriculum, practicum opportunity

Synaptic Training Institute

synaptic.institute
Established: 2020
Duration: 6 months
Format: online and in-person
Location: Portland, Oregon
Cost: $8500 but varies depending on which practicum location you choose
Advantages: rooted in holism, traditional wisdom, and science

Glossary

5-HT2A receptor: a receptor in the brain that is responsive to serotonin and is thought to play a pivotal role in causing the psychedelic experience

afterglow: a period of elevated and energetic mood with a relative freedom from concerns of the past, guilt, and anxiety

anxiolytic: an herb or pharmaceutical that reduces anxiety

ayahuasca: a brew made from a mixture of South American plants native to the Amazon basin, caapi (*Banisteriopsis caapi*) and chacruna (*Psychotria viridis*)

default mode network: the autopilot of the brain that is particularly active during wakeful rest; the part of the brain that seems to be impacted while on psilocybin

dissociative anesthetics: a class of hallucinogens that in the form of ketamine are now legal for the treatment of depression and major depressive disorder; with high enough dosage can cause separation from self and the world around you

dopamine: a brain neurotransmitter that is associated with the positive feelings of reward and outcome

empathogens: substances that promote feelings of empathy, awareness, and compassion

entheogen: a chemical substance, typically of plant origin, that is ingested to produce a non-ordinary state of consciousness for religious or spiritual purposes

magic truffle: a hardened mass of psilocybin mycelium; available in the Netherlands

major depressive disorder: a mental health disorder that is defined as persistent feelings of sadness and loss of interest in the daily activities of life

microdosing: taking small amounts of psilocybin that do not cause psychedelic experiences

neuroplasticity: the ability of neural networks in the brain to change through growth and reorganization

placebo: a substance lacking effect that is administered to the control group in a clinical trial or study

post-traumatic stress disorder (PTSD): a condition of persistent mental and emotional stress occurring as a result of injury or severe psychological shock, typically involving disturbance of sleep and constant vivid recall of the experience, with dulled responses to others and to the outside world

psilocin: the compound that psilocybin breaks down into after ingestion and which causes psychedelic effects

psychedelic: something that radically changes the consciousness

selective serotonin reuptake inhibitors (SSRIs): a class of pharmaceuticals prescribed for depression

serotonin: a brain neurotransmitter that is generally associated with happiness, focus, and love

set and setting: the mindset and environment of the participant for a psilocybin session

Notes

Introduction

1. Davis, A. K., Barrett, F. S., May, D. G., et al. 2020. Effects of psilocybin-assisted therapy on major depressive disorder. *JAMA Psychiatry* 78(5):481–489.

2. Parrington, John, *Redesigning Life: How genome editing will transform the world*, Oxford Press, 2016

Chapter 1

1. Cooke, J. 2021. Magic mushroom strain guide (100+ strains explained). *Tripsitter*. tripsitter.com/magic-mushrooms/strains

2. Fröhlich-Nowoisky, J., D. A. Pickersgill, V. R. Després, U. Pöschl. 2009. High diversity of fungi in air particulate matter. *Proceedings of the National Academy of Sciences USA* 106(31):12814–12819.

3. Guzmán, G., Yang Z. L. 2010. A new species of a bluing *Psilocybe* from Asia (Basidiomycota, Agaricales, Strophariaceae). *Sydowia* 62(2):185–189.

4. Lebowe, J. 2020. What are the differences among magic mushroom strains and their trips? *Merry Jane*. merryjane.com/culture/what-are-the-differences-among-magic-mushroom-strains-and-their-trips

Chapter 2

1. Johansen, P. Ø., Krebs, T. S. 2015. Psychedelics not linked to mental health problems or suicidal behavior: a population study. *Journal of Psychopharmacology* 29(3):270–279.

2. Schuster-Bruce, C. 2022. Terminally ill cancer patients in Canada received doses of the psychoactive substance found in 'magic' mushrooms after authorities eased rules. *Insider*. businessinsider.com/first-legal-magic-mushroom-psilocybin-canada-terminally-ill-cancer-patient-2022-4

3. Malone, T. C., Mennenga, S. E., Guss, J., et al. 2018. Individual experiences in four cancer patients following psilocybin-assisted psychotherapy. *Frontiers in Pharmacology* 9:256.

4. Gukasyan, N., Davis, A. K., Barrett, F. S., et al. 2022. Efficacy and safety of psilocybin-assisted treatment for major depressive disorder: Prospective 12-month follow-up. *Journal of Psychopharmacology* 36(2):151–158.

5. Carhart-Harris, R. L., Roseman, L. Bolstridge, M., et al. 2017. Psilocybin for treatment-resistant depression: fMRI-measured brain mechanisms. *Scientific Reports* 7:13187.

6. Naftulin, J. 2020. A Navy SEAL veteran with PTSD said a 'magic' mushroom trip put an end to his depression. *Insider*. insider.com/army-vet-with-ptsd-magic-mushroom-prevent-substanc-abuse-2020-11

7. Johnson, Matthew W., Garcia-Romeu, A., Griffiths, R. R. 2017. Long-term follow-up of psilocybin-facilitated smoking cessation. *American Journal of Drug and Alcohol Abuse* 43(1):55–60.

8. Bogenschutz, M. P., Ross, S., Bhatt, S., et al. 2022. Percentage of heavy drinking days following psilocybin-assisted psychotherapy vs placebo in the treatment of adult patients with alcohol use disorder. *JAMA Psychiatry* 79(10):953–962.

9. Bogenschutz, M. P., Podrebarac, S. K., Duane, J. H., et al. 2018. Clinical interpretations of patient experience in a trial of psilocybin-assisted psychotherapy for alcohol use disorder. *Frontiers in Pharmacology* 9:100.

10. Watts, A. 1970. Psychedelics and religious experience. In B. Aaronson and H. Osmond (eds.), *Psychedelics: The Uses and Implications of Hallucinogenic Drugs*. New York: Anchor Books, pp. 131–144.

11. Prochazkova, L., Lippelt, D. P., Colzato, L. S., et al. 2018. Exploring the effect of microdosing psychedelics on creativity in an open-label natural setting. *Psychopharmacology (Berlin)* 235(12):3401–3413.

Chapter 3

1. Rodríguez Arce, J. M., Winkelman, M. J. 2021. Psychedelics, sociality, and human evolution. *Frontiers in Psychology* 12:729425.

2. Ibid.

3. Garcia, S. A., Márquez, C. I. 2021. Cultivating positive health, learning, and community: the return of Mesoamerica's Quetzalcoatl and the Venus Star. *Genealogy* 5(2):53.

4. Berlant, S. 2005. The ethnomycological origin of Egyptian crowns and the esoteric underpinnings of Egyptian religion. *Journal of Ethnopharmacology* 102(2):275–288.

5. Keller, M. L. 2009. The ritual path of initiation into the Eleusinian Mysteries. *Rosicrucian Digest* 2:28–42.

6. Check out these ethnographic recordings of Maria Sabina: folkways.si.edu/maria-sabina/mushroom-ceremony-of-the-mazatec-indians-of-mexico/american-indian-sacred/music/album/smithsonian

7. Watts, A. 1970. Psychedelics and religious experience. In B. Aaronson and H. Oesmond (eds.), *Psychedelics: The Uses and Implications of Hallucinogenic Drugs*. New York: Anchor Books, pp. 131–144.

Chapter 4

1. Nutt, D. 2012.

Chapter 5

1. Johnson, M. W., Richards, W. A., Griffiths, R. R. 2008. Human hallucinogen research: guidelines for safety. *Journal of Psychopharmacology* 22(6):603–620.

2. Phelps, J. 2017. Developing guidelines and competencies for the training of psychedelic therapists. *Journal of Humanistic Psychology* 57(5):450–487.

3. Grof, S. 1980. *LSD Psychotherapy*. Alameda, CA: Hunter House.

4. Zohar, D. 2018. Spiritual intelligence: a new paradigm for collaborative action. Available via thesystemsthinker.com.

5. Maslow, A. 1971. *The Farther Reaches of Human Nature*. New York: Penguin, p. 269.

Chapter 6

1. Hartogsohn, I. 2021. Set and setting in the Santo Daime. *Frontiers in Pharmacology* 12:651037.

Chapter 9

1. Wasser, S. P. 2017. Medicinal mushrooms in human clinical studies. Part I. Anticancer, oncoimmunological, and immunomodulatory activities: a review. *International Journal of Medicinal Mushrooms* 19(4):279–317.

Chapter 10

1. Hutcheson, J. D., Setola, V., Roth, B. L., et al. 2011. Serotonin receptors and heart valve disease: it was meant 2B. *Pharmacology & Therapeutics* 132(2):146–157.

2. Hackl, B., Todt, H., Kubista, H., et al. 2022. Psilocybin therapy of psychiatric disorders is not hampered by hERG potassium channel–mediated cardiotoxicity. *International Journal of Neuropsychopharmacology* 25(4):280–282.

3. Becker, A. M., Holze, F., Grandinetti, T., et al. 2022. Acute effects of psilocybin after escitalopram or placebo pretreatment in a randomized, double-blind, placebo-controlled, crossover study in healthy subjects. *Clinical Pharmacology of Therapeutics* 111(4):886–895.

4. Dr. Erica Zelfand, ND. https://ericazelfand.com/video-combining-psilocybin-and-antidepressants-ssris-etc.

5. Malcolm, B., Thomas, K. 2022. Serotonin toxicity of serotonergic psychedelics. *Psychopharmacology (Berlin)* 239(6):1881–1891.

6. Gard, D. E., Pleet, M. M., Bradley, E. R., et al. 2021. Evaluating the risk of psilocybin for the treatment of bipolar depression: A review of the research literature and published case studies. *Journal of Affective Disorders Reports* 6:100240.

Chapter 11

1. Schmitz, G. P., Jain, M. K., Slocum, S. T., et al. 2022. 5-HT2A SNPs alter the pharmacological signaling of potentially therapeutic psychedelics. *ACS Chemical Neuroscience* 13(16):2386–2398.

2. Wojtas, A., Bysiek, A., Wawrzczak-Bargiela, A., et al. 2022. Effect of psilocybin and ketamine on brain neurotransmitters, glutamate receptors, DNA and rat behavior. *International Journal of Molecular Sciences* 23:6713.

Bibliography

Abramson, H. A., Hewitt, M. P., Lennard, H., et al. 1958. The stablemate concept of therapy as affected by LSD in schizophrenia. *Journal of Psychology* 45(1):75–84.

Aronson, J. K. 2016. Psilocybin. In *Meyler's Side Effects of Drugs*. 16th ed. New York: Elsevier, pp. 1048-1–51.

Arthur, J. 2003. *Mushrooms and Mankind*. Escondido, CA: The Book Tree.

Austin, P. 2023. The LSD psychedelic experience: best practices, set & setting. *Third Wave*. thethirdwave.co/set-setting-lsd/

Bear, M. F., Connors, B. W., Paradiso, M. A. 2020. *Neuroscience: Exploring the Brain*. Burlington, MA: Jones & Bartlett Learning.

The Beckley/Imperial Psychedelic Research Programme. beckleyfoundation.org/science/collaborations/the-beckley-imperial-psychedelic-research-programme/

Berlant, S. R. 2005. The entheomycological origin of Egyptian crowns and the esoteric underpinnings of Egyptian religion. *Journal of Ethnopharmacology* 102(2):275–288.

Bogadi, M., Kaštelan, S. 2021. A potential effect of psilocybin on anxiety in neurotic personality structures in adolescents. *Croatian Medical Journal* 62(5):528–530.

Bogenschutz, M. P., Forcehimes, A. A., Pommy, J. A., et al. 2015. Psilocybin-assisted treatment for alcohol dependence: a proof-of-concept study. *Journal of Psychopharmacology* 29(3):289–299.

Brand, D. S. 2021. The Stamets stack: Can microdosing really change your brain? *DoubleBlind Mag.* doubleblindmag.com/stamets-stack

Bronner, D. 2022. On entheogenic practitioner duties and privileges under Oregon's 109 Program. *Dr. Bronner's All One.* drbronner.com/all-one-blog/2022/04/entheogenic-practitioner-duties-and-privileges-under-oregons-109-program

Carhart-Harris, R. L., Muthukumaraswamy, S., Roseman, L., et al. 2016. Neural correlates of the LSD experience revealed by multimodal neuroimaging. *Proceedings of the National Academy of Sciences U.S.A.* 113(17):4853–4858.

Catlow, B. J., Song, S., Paredes, D. A., et al. 2013. Effects of psilocybin on hippocampal neurogenesis and extinction of trace fear conditioning. *Experimental Brain Research* 228(4):481–491.

Center for Behavioral Health Statistics and Quality. 2018. *The 2017 National Survey on Drug Use and Health: Detailed Tables.* Rockville, MD: Substance Abuse and Mental Health Services Administration. samhsa.gov/data/sites/default/files/cbhsq-reports/NSDUHDetailedTabs2017/NSDUHDetailedTabs2017.pdf

Cooke, J. 2021. Magic mushroom strain guide (100+ strains explained). *Tripsitter.* tripsitter.com/magic-mushrooms/strains/

Dorr, A. 2021. The history of psilocybin: magic mushrooms through the ages. *Mushroom Revival.* mushroomrevival.com/blogs/blog/the-history-of-psilocybin-magic-mushroom-use-through-the-ages

Ehrlich, B. 2017. LSD doc 'Sunshine Makers': what we learned. *Rolling Stone.* rollingstone.com/culture/culture-news/lsd-doc-sunshine-makers-what-we-learned-129705/

Eiden, L. E., Weihe, E. 2011. VMAT2: a dynamic regulator of brain monoaminergic neuronal function interacting with drugs of abuse. *Addiction Review* 1216(1):86–98.

Erowid. n.d. MDMA basics. *The Vaults of Erowid*. erowid.org/
chemicals/mdma/mdma_basics.shtml

Froese, T., Guzmán, G., Guzmán-Dávalos, L. 2016. On the origin of
the genus *Psilocybe* and its potential ritual use in ancient Africa and
Europe. *Economic Botany* 70(2):103–114.

Gartz, J. 1991. Further Investigations on psychoactive mushrooms of
the genera *Psilocybe*, *Gymnopilus* and *Conocybe*. *Annals of Museum
of Reverto* 7:265–274 museocivico.rovereto.tn.it/UploadDocs/748_
Annali71991_art13_gartz.pdf

Gartz, J. 1996. *Magic Mushrooms Around the World*. cdn.preterhuman.
net/texts/drugs/Magic.Mushrooms.Around.The.World.By.Jochen.
Gartz.pdf

Goldberg, S., Pace, B. T., Nicholas, C. R., et al. 2020. The experimental
effects of psilocybin on symptoms of anxiety and depression:
a meta-analysis. *Psychiatry Research* 284:112749.

Grant, R. 2018. Do trees talk to each other? *Smithsonian Magazine*.
smithsonianmag.com/science-nature/the-whispering-trees-
180968084/

Griego, T. 2020. *Wound Swimming: Healing with Psilocybin, Ceremonies
& Micro-dosing*. Self-published. Available at Amazon.

Griffiths, R. R., Johnson, M. W., Carducci, M. A., et al. 2016. Psilocybin
produces substantial and sustained decreases in depression and anxiety in patients with life-threatening cancer: a randomized double-blind
trial. *Journal of Psychopharmacology* 30(12):1181–1197.

Grob, C. S. 2002. *Hallucinogens*. Washington, DC: National Geographic
Books.

Guzman, G., Nixon, S., Ramirez-Guilles, F., et al. 2014. *Psilocybe* s. str.
(Agaricales, Strophariaceae) in Africa with description of a new species
from the Congo. *Sydowia* 66:434–453.

Hackl, B., Todt, H., Kubista, H., et al. 2022. Psilocybin therapy of psychiatric disorders is not hampered by hERG potassium channel–mediated cardiotoxicity. *International Journal of Neuropsychopharmacology* 25(4):280–282.

Halberstadt, A. L. 2018. *Behavioral Neurobiology of Psychedelic Drugs*. New York: Springer.

Hallifax, J. 2022. How to microdose psilocybin according to Paul Stamets. *Psychedelic Spotlight*. psychedelicspotlight.com/how-to-microdose-psilocybin-paul-stamets-the-stamets-stack

Hartney, E. 2023. What are psychedelic drugs? *Verywell Mind*. verywellmind.com/what-are-the-effects-of-hallucinogens-67500#toc-short-term-effects

Hartogsohn, I. 2017. Constructing drug effects: a history of set and setting. *Drug Science, Policy and Law*, 3:2050324516683325.

Hofmann, A. 2017. *LSD: My Problem Child:* Reflections on Sacred Drugs, Mysticism and Science. 4th ed. Santa Cruz, CA: Multidisciplinary Association for Psychedelic Studies.

Holewinski, B. 2018. Underground networking: the amazing connections beneath your feet. *National Forest Foundation*. nationalforests.org/blog/underground-mycorrhizal-network

Hutcheson, J. D., Setola, V., Roth, B. L., et al. 2011. Serotonin receptors and heart valve disease: it was meant 2B. *Pharmacology & Therapeutics* 132(2):146–157.

Isokauppila, T. 2017. *Healing Mushrooms*. New York: Avery.

Janikian, M. 2019. *Your Psilocybin Mushroom Companion*. New York: Simon and Schuster.

John Hopkins Medicine. 2014. 'Magic mushrooms' help long-time smokers quit. hopkinsmedicine.org/news/media/releases/magic_mushrooms_help_longtime_smokers_quit

Johnson, M. W., Garcia-Romeu, A., Griffiths, R. R. 2017. Long-term follow-up of psilocybin-facilitated smoking cessation. *The American Journal of Drug and Alcohol Abuse* 43(1):55–60.

Johnson, M. W., Griffiths, R. R., Hendricks, P. S., et al. 2018. The abuse potential of medical psilocybin according to the 8 factors of the Controlled Substances Act. *Neuropharmacology* 142:143–166.

Keremedchiev, S. 2016. Psychedelics: effects on the human brain and physiology. YouTube. youtube.com/watch?v=FyAgx_tzh80

Kimbrawification. 2018. The psychedelic experience: a manual based on the Tibetan Book of the Dead, games and game reality. *Hive*. hive.blog/philosophy/@kimbrawification/the-psychedelic-experience-a-manual-based-on-the-tibetan-book-of-the-dead-games-and-game-reality

Kowalski, K. 2019. What is transcendence? The top of Maslow's hierarchy of needs (+ visual). *Sloww*. sloww.co/transcendence-maslow

Labate, B. C., Cavnar, C. (eds.) 2021. *Psychedelic Justice:* Toward a Diverse and Equitable Psychedelic Culture. Santa Fe, NM: Synergetic Press.

Lane, C. 2022. A decisive blow to the serotonin hypothesis of depression. *Psychology Today*. psychologytoday.com/us/blog/side-effects/202207/decisive-blow-the-serotonin-hypothesis-depression

Leary, T. 1966. Programmed communication during experiences with DMT. *Psychedelic Review* Issue 8. deoxy.org/h_leary.htm

Leary, T., Metzner, R., Alpert, R. 2007. *The Psychedelic Experience: A Manual Based on the Tibetan Book of the Dead*. New York: Citadel Press.

Letcher, A. 2008. *Shroom:* A Cultural History of the Magic Mushroom. New York: Ecco.

Lhooq, M. 2021. Countdown to ecstasy: how music is being used in healing psychedelic trips. *The Guardian*. theguardian.com/music/2021/oct/22/countdown-to-ecstasy-how-music-is-being-used-in-healing-psychedelic-trips

MacBride, K. 2021. "Aharon said it was healing:" How psychedelic therapy was undermined by abuse. *Inverse*. inverse.com/mind-body/grossbard-bourzat-psychedelic-assisted-therapy-abuse/amp

Madsen, M. K., Fisher, P. M., Burmester, D., et al. 2019. Psychedelic effects of psilocybin correlate with serotonin 2A receptor occupancy and plasma psilocin levels. *Neuropsychopharmacology* 44(7):1328–1334.

Main, D. 2013. Mushrooms "make wind" to spread spores. *Livescience*. livescience.com/41492-mushrooms-make-wind.html

Mann, J. J. 1999. Role of the serotonergic system in the pathogenesis of major depression and suicidal behavior. *Neuropsychopharmacology* 21(2):99S–105S.

Mason, N. L., Kuypers, K. P. C., Reckweg, J. T., et al. 2021. Spontaneous and deliberate creative cognition during and after psilocybin exposure. *Translational Psychiatry* 11:209.

McKenna, A. 2020. *Psilocybin Mushrooms*. Self-published. Available at Amazon.

McNamara, S. 2022. *Blue Thumb: How to Grow Psilocybin Mushrooms at Home*. Self-published. Available at Amazon.

Mechura, S. 2015. Are mushrooms from outer space? *Explore Big Sky*. explorebigsky.com/are-mushrooms-from-outer-space/16984

Metzner, R. 2022. *Allies for Awakening:* Guidelines for Productive and Safe Experiences with Entheogens. El Verano, CA: Four Trees Press.

Microdosing Institute. Microdosing protocol. microdosinginstitute.com/how-to/microdosing-protocols

Miech, R., Johnston, L., O'Malley, P., et al. 2019. *Monitoring the Future National Survey Results on Drug Use, 1975–2018. Vol. 1. Secondary School Students.* Ann Arbor: University of Michigan.

Moore, C. 2020. What are the differences among magic mushroom strains and their trips? *Merry Jane.* merryjane.com/culture/what-are-the-differences-among-magic-mushroom-strains-and-their-trips

Multidisciplinary Association for Psychedelic Studies. 2017. David Nutt: psychedelic research, from brain imaging to policy reform. YouTube. youtube.com/watch?v=ZzepSK6Gzk8

Muraresku, B. C. 2020. *Immortality Key:* The Secret History of the Religion with No Name. New York: St. Martin's Press.

Naftulin, J. 2020. Listen: the playlist scientists used to unlock 'elevated states of consciousness' in people tripping on 'magic' mushrooms for a research study. *Insider.* insider.com/listen-psychedelic-playlist-researchers-use-to-reach-elevated-state-2020-11

Nichols, D. 2013. LSD neuroscience. YouTube. youtube.com/watch?v=LbUGRcuA16E

Nichols, D. 2017. Serotonin, and the past and future of LSD. *MAPS Bulletin.* maps.org/news-letters/v23n1/v23n1_p20-23.pdf

Orion, D. 2016. Achieving the "set" in set and setting: 4 principles to make the most of your psychedelic experience. *Psychedelic Times.* psychedelictimes.com/achieving-set-in-set-and-setting-4-principles-make-most-of-your-psychedelic-experience

Petri, G., Expert, P., Turkheimer, F., et al. 2014. Homological scaffolds of brain functional networks. *Journal of the Royal Society Interface* 11(101):20140873.

Pollan, M. 2015. The trip treatment. *The New Yorker.* newyorker.com/magazine/2015/02/09/trip-treatment

Pollan, M. 2019. *How to Change Your Mind*. New York: Penguin.

Powell, S. G. 2015. *Magic Mushroom Explorer*. New York: Park Street Press.

Presti, D. E. 2015. *Foundational Concepts in Neuroscience*. New York: W.W. Norton.

Prochazkova, L., Lippelt, D. P., Colzato, L. S., et al. 2018. Exploring the effect of microdosing psychedelics on creativity in an open-label natural setting. *Psychopharmacology (Berlin)* 235(12):3401–3413.

Psychedelic Support. 2022. Psilocybin and antidepressants: what patients need to know. YouTube. youtube.com/watch?v=v1r5u71JT2k

Reneman, L., Endert, E., de Bruin, K., et al. 2002. The acute and chronic effects of MDMA ("ecstasy") on cortical 5-HT2A receptors in rat and human brain. *Neuropsychopharmacology* 26(3):387–396.

Rex, E. 2022. Fake drug guru & serial plagiarist uses woman's writing to bag his latest career. *Medium*. erica-rex.medium.com/my-original-published-work-was-plagiarized-by-a-famous-white-male-writer-now-he-owns-the-topic-19d0e9f5391e

Richards, W. A. 2015. *Sacred Knowledge*. New York: Columbia University Press.

Rogers, R. D. 2020. *Medicinal Mushrooms: The Human Clinical Trials*. Self-published. Available at Amazon.

Rogers, R. D. 2021. *Psilocybin Mushrooms: The Magic, Science and Research*. Self-published. Available at Amazon.

Rosegrant, J. 1976. The impact of set and setting on religious experience in nature. *Journal for the Scientific Study of Religion* 15(4):301.

Ruck, C. A. 2009. *Mushrooms, Myth, and Mithras*. San Francisco: City Lights Publishers.

Rupp, M. 2018. Psychedelic drugs and the serotonergic system. *Sapiensoup*. sapiensoup.com/serotonin

Samorini, G. n.d. The hallucinogenic mushrooms of the Sahara. (In Italian.) samorini.it/archeologia/africa/funghi-allucinogeni-teste-rotonde/

Schuster-Bruce, C. 2022. Terminally ill cancer patients in Canada received doses of the psychoactive substance found in 'magic' mushrooms after authorities eased rules. *Insider*. businessinsider.com/first-legal-magic-mushroom-psilocybin-canada-terminally-ill-cancer-patient-2022-4

Shewan, D., Dalgarno, P., Reith, G. 2000. Perceived risk and risk reduction among ecstasy users: the role of drug, set, and setting. *International Journal of Drug Policy* 10(6):431–453.

Smith, D. G. 2022. More people are microdosing for mental health. But does it work? *New York Times*. nytimes.com/2022/02/28/well/mind/microdosing-psychedelics.html

Smith, P. 2017. Psychedelics and heart risk: Can LSD cause a heart attack? *Third Wave*. thethirdwave.co/psychedelics-heart-risk

Sodhi, M. S. K., Sanders-Bush, E. 2004. Serotonin and brain development. *International Review of Neurobiology* 59:111–174.

Stamets, P. 1996. *Psilocybin Mushrooms of the World*. San Francisco: Ten Speed Press.

Stamets, P. 2014. Mycologist Paul Stamets explains how mushrooms can save the Earth. YouTube. youtube.com/watch?v=imVh-KfH2hI

Stolaroff, M. J. 2020. *The Secret Chief Revealed*. 2nd ed. Santa Cruz, CA: Multidisciplinary Association for Psychedelic Studies.

Strassman, R. 2022. *Psychedelic Handbook*. New York: Simon and Schuster.

Strickland, J. C., Garcia-Romeu, A., & Johnson, M. W. 2021. Set and setting: a randomized study of different musical genres in supporting psychedelic therapy. *ACS Pharmacology & Translational Science* 4(2):472–478.

Sweat, N. W., Bates, L. W., Hendricks, P. S. 2016. The associations of naturalistic classic psychedelic use, mystical experience, and creative problem solving. *Journal of Psychoactive Drugs* 48(5):344–350.

Thoricatha, W. 2015. The building blocks of life: Kary Mullis and Francis Crick's psychedelic breakthrough. *Psychedelic Times*. psychedelictimes.com/building-blocks-life-karry-mullis-francis-crick-psychedelic-breakthrough/

Toomy, D. 2016. Exploring how and why trees 'talk' to each other. *Yale E360*. e360.yale.edu/features/exploring_how_and_why_trees_talk_to_each_other

Tripson, D. M. 2020. *Magic Mushroom User's Guide*. Self-published. Available at Amazon.

Urban, T. 2017. Neuralink and the brain's magical future. *Wait But Why*. waitbutwhy.com/2017/04/neuralink.html#part2

Wasson, R. G., Ruck, C., Hofmann, A. 2008. *The Road to Eleusis*. Berkeley: North Atlantic Books.

Welcome to Microdosing Psychedelics.com. Microdosingpsychedelics.com

Whitaker-Azmitia, P. 1999. The discovery of serotonin and its role in neuroscience. *Neuropsychopharmacology* 21(2):2S-8S.

Whitehurst, L. 2016. My life was a wreck. WOAI. news4sanantonio.com/news/nation-world/my-life-was-a-wreck-veteran-uses-magic-mushrooms-to-treat-ptsd

Williams, M. T. 2020. *Managing Microaggressions*. New York: Oxford University Press.

Winkelman, M. J. 2019. *Advances in Psychedelic Medicine*. Santa Barbara, CA: ABC-CLIO.

World Health Organization. 1958. Ataractic and hallucinogenic drugs in psychiatry. *World Health Organization Technical Report* 152. apps.who.int/iris/bitstream/handle/10665/40410/WHO_TRS_152.pdf

Zafeiriou, D., Ververi, A., Vargiami, E. 2009. The serotonergic system: its role in pathogenesis and early developmental treatment of autism. *Current Neuropharmacology* 7(2):150–157.

Zefland, E. 2022. Combining psilocybin and antidepressants (SSRIs, etc.). ericazelfand.com/video-combining-psilocybin-and-antidepressants-ssris-etc/

Zohar, D. 2016. Spiritual intelligence: a new paradigm for collaborative action. *The Systems Thinker*. thesystemsthinker.com/spiritual-intelligence-a-new-paradigm-for-collaborative-action

Index

4-AcO-DET, 65

23&Me (ancestry test), 175

1960s, about, 36, 48, 66–67

A

Abram, David, 72

abuse of power, warnings against, 96–100

acceptance and commitment therapy (ACT), 132

Acetyl-l-carnitine, 177

Acid Test (Shroder), 42

adaptogens, 159

addiction treatment, 22, 43–46

addictive potential of psychoactive drugs, 18, 79, 81

Africa, history of psilocybin in, 59–60

"aha moments," 36

Albino A+ (*Psilocybe cubensis* strain), 28–29

alcohol and alcohol abuse, 43, 44–46, 79, 114

Alcoholics Anonymous, 44, 45

alert quietism, state of, 121

alkaline phosphatase, 179

alkaloids, 26–27, 65

allies, attendance at psilocybin sessions, 111–112

Alpert, Richard (Ram Dass), 66, 70, 116

alpha waves, 83

Amanita muscaria, 62

Amanita mushrooms, 30

America, history of psilocybin in, 63–69. *See also* Mexico

American Psychedelic Practitioners Association, 96

ancestral lineage healing, 141

anorexia nervosa, 44

antioxidants, 156, 157, 158, 178

anxiety during psilocybin sessions, 119

anxiety treatment, 17, 38–41, 45–46, 150

archetypes and symbols seen in altered states, 122

Artha (second aim of The Purusharthas), 34

arthritis treatment, 157

Atropa belladonna, 44

attendants for psilocybin therapy. *See* facilitators for psilocybin therapy

Australia, psychedelic mushroom use in, 63
ayahuasca, 72, 122
Aztec culture, psilocybin use in,
57

B
bad trips, 125
baeocystin (alkaloid), 27
Bardo Thodol, 116–118
barriers to use, 50–51
bathroom, visiting, 120
B complex, 177
The Beatles, 67
The Beeman, 122
belladonna, 44
Berlant, Stephen, 60
Berry, Wendell, on herbalism, 21
beta waves, 83
biochemical pathways, 173–174
BIPOC communities, 97, 98
bipolar disorder, 170
Bird, Christopher, 29
block tactics, 143
blood pressure, high, treatment
for, 158
blood tests, 174
blood thinner cautions, 158
Board of Psychedelic Medicine
and Therapies, 187
Book of the Dead (Egypt), 60
Book of the Dead, Tibetan,
116–118

brain function and chemistry,
effects of psilocybin on,
77–84
brain waves, 83
British Isles, history of psilocybin
in, 61–62
Burton, Mr. (patient), 166

C
caffeine, 79
California Institute of Integral
Studies, 11, 91, 184
cancer patients, treatment for,
38–41, 67, 69, 157, 158, 159
Capacha culture, 56
capitalism, 51, 75
cardiac disease risk, 171
cardiac ion channels, 165
cardiologists, 166
Carhart-Harris, Robin, 42
catechol-o-methyltransferase
(enzyme), 176
Causes, Identify and Treat the
(naturopathic tenet), 163
cave art, 59–60, 62, 63, 123
Cavnar, Clancy, 75
Centella asiatica, 160
Centers for Disease Control and
Prevention, 44
Central America, psilocybin
history in, 56–59
Certificate in Psychedelic Training and Research, 184

Chacruna Institute, 75

chaga mushrooms, 158

chamomile tea, 180

changes, making big, after
    sessions, 126

chikhai bardo phase, 116–117

cholesterol treatment, 156, 158

chonyid bardo phase, 117

Chrissy (cancer patient),
    40–41

cigarette smoking, stopping of,
    43–44

citizen science, 152, 162

clairsentience, increased, 108

clergy and religious leaders as
    facilitators, 101

clinical trials, 69, 130–131, 151

clothing for psilocybin sessions,
    114

Codex Mexicanus I, 56

Codex Vindobonensis, 63

cofactors, 174, 175, 177

cognitive behavioral therapy
    (CBT), 132

colonialism and colonialist
    ideals, 56, 58, 75

Colorado (state), 86

colorblind patients, and micro-
    dosing, 150

comedown period, 113–114,
    124–125

comfort in psilocybin sessions,
    115, 119–120

COMPASS Pathways (pharma-
    ceutical and biotechnology
    company), 69

connection, finding, 10, 19,
    36–37, 40, 46–48, 52, 65,
    94, 149. See also nature,
    connection to

consciousness, rising to, 118–119,
    121–122

Cordyceps mushrooms, 153, 157

Cordyceps sinensis, 157

Coriolus versicolor, 156, 158

cortisol, 139

countertransfernce and trans-
    ference, warning against,
    99–100

creativity, increasing, 48–50

cultural appropriation, 56, 65,
    69–75

curanderas, 30, 58, 64, 88

The Cut (podcast), 99

CYPP450 (enzyme), 176

cytochrome enzymes, 176

D

Datura wrightii, 122

Davis, Alan K., 17

death, acceptance of,
    38–41, 65

default mode network, 81–83,
    109, 123

delinquents, 35

depression and depression
treatment
author's experiences with, 136
healing with psilocybin, 33,
38, 41
research on, 17–18, 42, 69
and seritonin, 78
and SSRIs, 167–168
"Developing Guidelines and
Competencies for the Training
of Psychedelic Therapists"
(Phelps), 91
Dharma (first aim of The Purusharthas), 34
diabetes treatment, 158, 159
diet, importance of, 178
discomfort in psilocybin
sessions, 119–120
disorienting experiences, 87
Docere (naturopathic tenet),
163
Doctor as Teacher (naturopathic
tenet), 163
doors, 14
The Doors of Perception (Huxley),
70
dopamine, 78, 79, 180
dosages for psilocybin therapy,
16–17, 109–111, 165, 168.
See also microdosing and
microdoses
drinking of water and other
liquids. See hydration

driving and psilocybin sessions, 124
drug interactions, potential,
167–168
Drug Policies and the Politics
of Drugs in the Americas
(ed. by Labate, Cavner, and
Rodrigues), 75
Druid culture, 62
Dylan, Bob, 67

E

eating, before. during, and after
psilocybin sessions, 113–114,
124, 125, 178
Egyptian Book of the Dead, 60
The Electric Kool-Aid Acid Test
(Wolfe), 66
electrocardiogram (ECG), 165
electroencephalogram (EEG), 83
electrolytes, 180
The Eleusinian Mysteries
ceremony, 61
Eliade, Mircea, 55
elimination pathway, 179
emotions, considered "bad," 133
empathy, 91–92, 108, 140
enjoyment and pleasure aims, 34
enlightenment aims, 36–37, 46,
64, 66, 67
entheogens, 15, 16. See also
psychedelics
environment, connection to,
47–48

epigenetics, 175–176

epilepsy and other seizure disorders, 166

erinacines, 157

ethical integrity, role of, 95–100

ethics, psychedelic, 183–188

ethics board, 185–187

European Americans, and psilocybin, 69–72

Evenki language, 54

eye movement desensitization and reprocessing (EMDR), 132, 133

eyeshades as part of psilocybin sessions, 113, 114

F

facilitators for psilocybin therapy

about, 85–104

and abuse of power, 96–100

clergy and religious leaders as, 101

and dosages, 109

and ethics, 95–100

and inner healers, 142–143

and integration sessions, 130–131

and power differentials, 96–99

pre-session appointments with, 89–91, 108, 128

professional backgrounds, 100–102

role of empathy, 91–92

role of trust, 92–93

selection of, 85–87, 89–96, 100–104, 126, 133, 187–188

and sense of humor, 95

and session comfort, 109, 115

sitters as, 102

and spiritual intelligence, 94–95

traditional, 88

training of, 88

Fadiman, James, 49, 70, 123, 151–153, 161

Fadiman Protocol, 152–153

Father Triglav (god as mountain), 73

FDA, 69, 186

Ferris wheel symbol, 40

fiber intake, 178

First, Do No Harm (naturopathic tenet), 163

flashbacks, 170

flavonoids, 26

flowers as part of psilocybin sessions, 114

fly agaric mushroom, 62

focal points, 160–161

folate, 177

four aims of human life, 34

Frohlich-Nowoisky, Janine, 23

functional mushrooms, 156–161, 179–180

fungi, 21–31

Fungi Perfect (company), 156

Furst, Peter T., 58

G

Ganoderma lucidum, 156, 159

Gard, David E., 170

genetic factors, 175–176

ginger, 180

Ginsberg, Allen, 66

God, experiences of, 46, 65

go-go-go state, 148

Golden Teacher (*Psilocybe cubensis* strain), 28, 29

Good Chemistry (Holland), 173

Good Friday experiment, 46, 67, 70

gotu kola, 160

The Grateful Dead, 67

gratitude, 74, 94, 102, 125

Greece, history of psilocybin in, 61

Grey, Alex, 50, 123

Grey, Allyson, 50

Griego, Tiana, 110

Griffiths, Roland R., 69

Grifola frondosa, 153, 159

Grof, Stan, 59, 70, 93

Guanyin (goddess), 122

Guzmán Huerta, Gastón, 56, 58, 70

H

hallucinations during psilocybin sessions, 121, 122–123

hallucinogen persisting perception disorder, 170

hallucinogens. *See* psychedelics

Hallucinogens and Culture (Furst), 58

halos, 171

Harper's Bazaar, 147

Hartogsohn, Ido, 106

headphones as part of psilocybin sessions, 113, 114

healing and health, 106, 125, 127–130, 137, 141–143, 175–176, 181

healing crisis (term), 125

The Healing Power of Nature (naturopathic tenet), 163

health professionals as facilitators, 101

heart damage risk, 164–166

Heffter Research Institute, 69

clinical trials through, 130

Heim, Roger, 65

henbane, 44

hen of the woods, 159

The Herbal Apothecary (Pursell), 179

herbalism (plant medicine), 21, 26–27, 160–161, 186

herbal supplements, 178

hericenones, 157

Hericium erinaceus, 153, 156

Hernández de Toledo, Francisco, 57

heroic doses, 110

Heroic Hearts Project website, 43

hippies, 35

Historia de las cosas de Nueva España (Sahagún), 57

A History of Medicine (Prioreschi), 151

Hofmann, Albert, 14–15, 61, 65, 70

Holland, Julie, 173

hopelessness, treatment for, 38–39

hospices, 38–41

Hubbard, Alfred Matthew, 107

Huffington Post, 147

Humongous Fungus, 25

Huxley, Aldous, 70

hybidization, defined, 28

hydration, 114, 125, 126, 177, 178, 180

Hyoscyamus niger, 44

hyphae, 22, 24, 25

I

Identify and Treat the Causes (naturopathic tenet), 163

immune system support, 158, 159, 179–180

Imperial College London, 42, 83

Indocybin (psicilocybin product for research), 28, 65

inflammation, reducing, 158, 167–168, 177, 178–179

inner healers, 141–143, 144

Inocybe (genus), 23. *See also* psilocybin

Inonotus obliquus, 158

Insider (magazine), 43

integration and integration therapists, 41–42, 43, 118, 125, 127–133, 171

internal family systems therapy, 132–133

internal family systems therapy (IFS therapy), 139

iPhone, 49

Ireland, history of psilocybin in, 61–62

isolation process, 29

J

Jobs, Steve, 49–50

Johns Hopkins University, 17, 38, 39, 41, 44, 69, 130

Johnson, Matthew W., 86

Journal of the American Medical Association, 17

journals and journaling, 115, 121, 125, 130, 155, 177

Jung, Carl, 138

Jungian therapy, 135

K

Kama (third aim of The Puru-sharthas), 34

Kaye, Walter H., 44

Kuske, Chad, 43

kykeon, 61

L

Labate, Beatriz Caiuby, 75

lavender, oral, 177

Leary, Timothy, 14, 36, 66, 68, 70, 116–117

LeBaron, Darren (Darren Springer), 23, 59, 60

legalities, 86, 130–131

Leiden University, 49

Letcher, Andy, 62, 84

Leuner, Hanscarl, 103

Lewis-Williams, David, 123

Lexapro, 168

LGBTQIA+ communities, 98

liberty cap mushrooms, 62

Life magazine, 14, 28, 64, 65

lineage holders, 53, 54, 106–107, 109, 187

lion's mane mushrooms, 153–154, 156–157, 161

liver damage risks, 166

liver support, 159, 179

"living well" concept, 183–184

Lobelia inflata, 120

love, feelings of infinite, 19

LSD. *See also* psychedelics

　about, 48

　author's experiences with, 10

　books about, 42, 147

　Chrissy and, 40

　in documentary, 48

　Hofmann and, 14–15, 65

　Hubbard and, 107

　Jobs on, 49–50

　Mullis on, 50

　synthesized nature of, 72

　use of in 1960s, 48, 66

　Wilson and, 44

　Wolfe and, 66–67

L-tyrosine, 180

Lynch, Ben, 175

M

Magic Mushroom Explorer (Powell), 37, 47

magic mushrooms. *See also* psilocybin

　about, 25–31, 171

　books and articles, 14, 37, 47, 62, 64, 84

　nausea and, 120

　negative messaging, 21–22, 35

　and outer space theory, 23

　terminally-ill patient on, 38

　traditions surrounding, 56, 57

magnesium, 177

maitake mushrooms, 153, 159

Malheur National Forest (US), 25

Mangini, Mary, 114

MAOIs (monoamine oxidase inhibitors), 169–170

MAPS (Multidisciplinary Association for Psychedelic Studies), 17, 43, 130, 140, 186

Mark (alcohol addiction trial subject), 45–46

Martinez-Cruz, Paloma, 56, 58, 75

Maryland Psychiatric Research Center, 67, 68

Maslow, Abraham, 94

Mayan culture, psilocybin use in, 57–58

Mazatec people and culture, 29–30, 58, 64–65, 73

McKenna, Terence, 23, 70, 125

MDMA, 17, 43, 138, 140, 166

Measure 109 (Oregon), 86

medical doctors (MDs), 97

medical model of psilocybin use
  and dosages, 109
  and ethics, 186–187
  facilitator role in, 85–104
  and the inner healer, 142
  psychedelics within, 14, 18
  setting for, 106–107, 108–109
  terminology for, 35
  traditional facilitators in, 88

medicinal mushrooms, 156–161, 179–180

Medicinal Mushrooms (Rogers), 159

medicine-making process, 29–30

medicine people, 54

mental health contraindications, 170, 171

mental health issues, treatment of, 22, 37, 41–46, 52, 78–79, 152

Mesoamerica, psilocybin history in, 56–59

Mesoamerican and American Indians, use of psychedielics by, 63–64

metabolic pathway, 173

methylation, 177

Metzner, Ralph, 70, 116, 121

Mexico
  cave art in, 60
  ceremonies in, 107
  psilocybin history in, 56–59, 64–65
  and psychedelic tourism, 66

Michael (depression trial participant), 42

microdosing and microdoses
  about, 17, 147–155, 162
  book about, 147
  creating record of, 154–155
  functional mushrooms, 160–161
  vs. macrodoses, 150
  in research, 49

mindset. *See* set and setting

Mithoefer, Annie, 140

Mithoefer, Michael, 140, 170

Mixtec writings, 56

modern life, 147–148

Moksha (fourth aim of The Purusharthas), 34

monoamine oxidase inhibitors (MAOIs), 169–170

mother trees, 24

Mullis, Kary, 50

Multidisciplinary Association for Psychedelic Studies (MAPS), 17, 43, 130, 140, 186

mushrooms, 55–56, 62, 156–161, 179–180. *See also* magic mushrooms

Mushrooms, Myth & Mithras (Ruck), 16

music, 95, 109, 112–113

mutations, 28–29, 176

mycelia, 21, 22, 23, 24–25, 26

mycorrhizal networks, 22–24, 26

mystical experiences, 16. *See also* enlightenment aims

N

N-acetyl cysteine, 176

Nahuatl (language), 57

Na-R-ALA, 177

National Institute of Mental Health, 17

nature, connection to, 47–48, 72, 124–125

Nature, The Healing Power of (naturopathic tenet), 163

Nature magazine, 161

naturopathic physicians

and dosages, 150

and evaluation of health, 27

and healing crises, 125

and the inner healer, 142

and microdosing functional mushrooms, 160–161

oaths taken, 163

objectives of, 80

and power differentials, 98

and role of Nature in healing, 25, 163

and session preparation, 173, 174

nausea, reducing, 120, 180

neocortex, 83

nervines, 180

nervousness, combating, 178, 180

neurogenesis, 153–154

neuronal repatterning, 80–81

neuroplasticity, 167

neurotransmitters, 77–79

New Yorker magazine, 38

The New York Times, 147

niacin, 67, 153–154, 161

Nichols, David E., 68, 123

norbaeocystin (alkaloid), 27

North America, history of psilocybin in, 63–69

nutrient deficiencies, 173–174

O

Oaxaca (Mexico), 58, 64–65, 71

ocean images, and psilocybin sessions, 123–124

Olmecs, history of, 56

On Becoming a Person (Rogers), 91

Oregon (state)

capitalism in, 51

facilitators and training in, 22, 88, 185

proposed state exam, 187

psilocybin status in, 35, 86, 110

Oregon Psilocybin Advisory Board, 187

Osiris, 60

Osmond, Humphry, 16

Ötzi (a.k.a. the Iceman), 63

outer space, 23, 31

oxalate content, 158

P

Pahnke, Walter, 46, 67, 70

Pangaea theory, 55

panspermia, 23

parenting, microdosing and, 147–148, 149

Paul (author's patient), 80–81

PCR (polymerase chain reaction), 50

persistent psychosis, 170–171

Peter (patient), 143

peyote, 72

Phelps, Janis, 71, 91

photosynthate, 24

physical distractions. *See* block tactics

physical risks of psilocybin therapy, 164–166

physical symptoms during psilocybin sessions, 119–120, 142–143, 144

physicians' oaths, 163–164

picture books, use of in psilocybin sessions, 114, 118

PiHKAL (A. and A. Shulgin), 71

placebo effect, and microdosing, 161

plant communication, 22–24

Plant Medicines, Healing, and Psychedelic Science (ed. by Labate and Cavner), 75

pleasure and enjoyment aims, 34

Pollan, Michael, 38

polymerase chain reaction (PCR), 180

post-traumatic stress disorder (PTSD), treating, 22, 42–43, 129

Powell, Simon G,, 37, 47, 71

power differentials, warning against, 96–99

Praevenic (naturopathic tenet), 164

presence, 148

pre-session meetings with facilitator, 89–91, 92, 109, 115, 128, 130

Prevention (naturopathic tenet), 164

Primum non nocere (naturopathic tenet), 163

Prioreschi, Plinio, 151

problem-solving ability, increasing, 48–50

Procházková, Luisa, 49
professional backgrounds of
    facilitators, 100–102, 185
protectors, 139, 140, 145
protocols for microdosing,
    151–155
psilocin (alkaloid), 26–27, 65, 78,
    165
Psilocybe (genus). *See also* magic
    mushrooms
  about, 21
  isolation of parts, 65
  locations of, 26, 55, 58, 66, 74
  and outer space theory, 23
  strains of, 30
  therapeutic mushrooms as,
    25–27
Psilocybe aztecorum, 57
Psilocybe cubensis, 28–30, 166
Psilocybe hispanica, 63
Psilocybe mexicana, 57
Psilocybe natalensis, 59
Psilocybe semilanceata, 62
Psilocybe zapotecorum symbol-
    ism, 56
psilocybin. *See also* psychedelics
  about, 31
  cardiotoxic potential of, 165
  as a door, 14
  and empathy, 139
  and European Americans, 56
  genetic factors and, 175–176
  history and traditions of, 53–76

  important people, 66, 70–71
  isolation of, 27–28
  lineage holders for, 53, 54,
    106–107, 109, 187
  negative messaging about,
    50–51
  research on, 17–18
  safety of, 51
  in Stamets Protocol, 153–154,
    161
  use of in 1960s, 66
psilocybin (alkaloid), 26–27, 65
psilocybin therapy/sessions
  about, 105–126
  and ancestral lineage healing,
    141
  barriers to use of, 50–51
  cost of, 51
  deaths, 166
  dosages for, 16–17, 109–111, 165,
    168. *See also* microdosing and
    microdoses
  facilitator role in, 74, 85–104
  hydration after, 180
  microdosing and, 147–162
  and naturopathic physicians,
    164
  possible long-lasting effects,
    170–171
  potential risks, 164–171
  and power differentials, 96–99
  preparation for, 173–180
  reasons for, 33–52, 140

reducing nausea during, 180
and shadow work, 145
solo psychedelic sessions, 103
and SSRIs, 167
supplements in month before, 176–177
psychedelic ethics, 183–188
The Psychedelic Experience (Leary, Metzner, and Alpert), 116
The Psychedelic Explorer's Guide (Fadiman), 152
Psychedelic Justice (ed. by Labate and Cavner), 75
psychedelics
about, 31
and ancestral lineage healing, 141
author's experiences with, 9–11
in documentary, 48
as entheogens, 15, 16
history of, 14–15, 51
important people, 9
and increases in creativity, 49–50
microdosing and, 147
negative messaging, 21–22, 35, 68
research. *See* research into psychedelics
term defined, 16
and trauma patterns, 139

psychedelic therapy, 175–176, 187. *See also* medical model of psilocybin use; psilocybin therapy/sessions; psychedelics; *and specific substance names*
psychedelic tourism, 66, 75
psychoactive drugs, 79–81. *See also* psychedelics
psychotherapy, used in conjunction with psolocybin therapy, 41, 44
PTSD (post-traumatic stress disorder), treating, 22, 42–43, 129
Puharich, Andrija, 65
purging, 120
Pursell, J. J., 179
The Purusharthas (Hindu philosophy), 34–36

Q
QT wave, 165
Queen Toloache, 122
Quetzalcoatl, 56

R
racial biases in history of psychedelics, 51, 72
Ram Dass (Richard Alpert). *See* Alpert, Richard (Ram Dass)
Ray, Thomas S., 79
reaffirming statements, discussion of in pre-session appointments, 90

A Really Good Day (Waldman), 147

reasons for psilocybin therapy, 33–52

record creation, for microdosing, 154–155

reentry period. *See* comedown period

regulating bodies, lack of, 96

regulating of psychedelics, 186–187

reishi mushrooms, 156, 159

research into psychedelics
about, 15–18
in Africa, 59, 60
and creatiivity, 49
and default mode network, 83
and dosages, 109–110, 111
funding for, 68–69
and heart effects, 165
history of, 34, 67
and mental health, 37, 40, 41–43, 170
musical playlists for, 112
and R. G. Wasson article, 64–65
and risks, 164, 165, 168
and set and setting, 106

respect and ethics, 183–188

rest, importance of, 178

Richards, Bill
about, 71
and research, 68–69, 170
and Roquet, 59

Sacred Knowledge, 67
on sessions, 114
on sitters, 103
on spelling, 48
on trauma, 141

Richardson, Allan, 64

The Road to Eleusis (R. G. Wasson, Hofmann, and Ruck), 61

Rodrigues, Thiago, 75

Rodríguez Arce, José Manuel, 55

Rogers, Carl R., 91

Rogers, Richard Dale, 159

Roquet, Salvador, 58–59

roses as part of psilocybin sessions, 114, 126

Ruck, Carl A. P., 16, 61, 71

Rumi, 114

S

Sabina, María, 53, 64, 71, 73

sacred datura, 122

Sacred Knowledge (Richards), 67

safety considerations, 87, 89, 95, 96–100, 115, 128, 184–185

Sahagún, Bernardino de, 57

Sahara Desert, cave art in, 59–60

Salvia divinorum, 58

Sand, Nicholas, 48

Sandoz (pharmaceutical company), 28, 65

Saunders, Cicely, 39

schizophrenia, 170

Schultes, Richard, 53

Schwartz, Richard C., 133

scientific research. *See* research into psychedelics

Scully, Tim, 48

The Secret Life of Plants (Tompkins and Bird), 29

"Seeking the Magic Mushroom" (R. G. Wasson article), 14, 71

self-talk, negative, 136

Selva Pascuala cave (Spain), 63

sense of humor, role of, 95

serotonin 5-HT2AR gene, 176

serotonin agonists, 42

serotonin and serotonin receptors, 78–79, 150–151, 165, 167–168

serotonin reuptake inhibitors (SSRIs), 167–168, 171

serotonin syndrome, 169–170

serpents, 124

Sessa, Ben, 71

set and setting
  about, 105–109
  facilitator role in, 86, 87, 91, 95
  impact on pcilocybin experience, 30, 87
  and long-lasting effects from psilocybin session, 171
  and shadow self, 140

shadow self, 128, 135–145

Shamanism (Eliade), 55

shamans and shamanism, 54–55, 72

Shroder, Tom, 42

Shroom (Letcher), 62, 84

Shulgin, Alexander "Sasha," 71

Shulgin, Ann, 71

Shuman, Andrea, 160–161

sidpa bardo phase, 117–118

silence, at psilocybin sessions, 113, 119

Simard, Suzanne, 23, 24

single nucleotide polymorphism (SNP), 175, 176

sitters as facilitators, 102

sleep, importance of, 178

Slovenia, 73

SNP (single nucleotide polymorphism), 175, 176

Solie, Kathryn, 61

solo psychedelic sessions, 103

somatic work, 132, 133

South America, history of psilocybin in, 63–69

The Spell of the Sensuous (Abram), 72

spiritual enlightenment, 36–37, 46, 64, 66, 67

spiritual growth, 46

spiritual intelligence, role of, 94–95

spores, 22, 24–25

Springer, Darren (Darren Le Barron), 23, 59, 60

SSRIs (serotonin reuptake inhibitors), 167–168, 171

Stamets, Paul, 25–26, 47, 71, 151, 153–154, 156

Stamets Protocol, 153–154

Stamets Stack, 153, 161

St. Christopher's Hospice, 39

St. Paul's Monastery (Greece), 52

stress, treatment of, 80–81

suicidal behaviors, 37

The Sunshine Makers (documentary), 48

symbols and archetypes seen in altered states, 122

T

talking, 119, 136

talk therapy, 86, 92, 95, 132, 145

tannins, 26

Tasma, David, 39

tenets of patient care, 163–164

Teonanacatl, 122

teotlnanácatl, 57

terminally ill cancer patients, treatment for. See cancer patients, treatment for

testimonies, 18–19

Tezcatlipoca, 56

therapists, 97–98, 101

This Is Your Mind on Plants (Pollan), 38

Thurman, Howard, 67

The Tibetan Book of the Dead, 116–118

TiHKAL (A. and A. Shulgin), 71

Tin-Tazarift (Algerian caves), 60

Tolle causam (naturopathic tenet), 163

Tolle totum (naturopathic tenet), 163–164

Tompkins, Peter, 29

touch, discussion of in pre-session appointments, 89–90

tracers, 150

traditional model of psilocybin use

ceremonies, 102, 106

and dosages, 109

microdosing and, 151

setting for, 106–107, 108

and use of music, 112

trails, 171

transcendence, 94–95

transference and countertransference, warnings against, 99–100

transpersonal therapy, 132

trauma and trauma work

about, 136–137

and ancestral lineage healing, 141

healing from, 33, 42, 133

as part of integration, 131

and protectors, 139

psychedelic therapy and, 140, 141–143

and rising to consciousness, 121–122

triggers, 26, 51, 99–100, 128, 137, 143–144, 148

"The Trip Treatment" (Pollan article), 38

trust, role of, 92–93

turkey tail mushrooms, 158

type 2 diabetes treatment, 158

U

uncomfortable feelings in psilocybin sessions, 119–120

University of California San Diego Eating Disorders Center, 44

V

veladas, 58

Veteran Voices, 43

Visionary Art movement, 50

visions during psilocybin sessions, 121, 122–123

Vis medicatrix naturae (naturopathic tenet), 163

visuals during psilocybin sessions, 121, 122–123

vitamin B$_3$ (niacin), 67, 153–154, 161

vitamin B$_6$, 177

vitamin B$_{12}$, 174, 177

Vitamin C, 177

W

wakeful rest or daydreaming state, 81–82

Waldman, Ayelet, 147

The War on Drugs, 15, 26, 35

Wasser, Solomon P., 156

Wasson, R. Gordon, 14, 28, 53, 61, 64–65, 71, 73

Wasson, Valentina, 64

water, drinking, and other liquids. *See* hydration

Watts, Alan, 46

Western model of psilocybin use. *See* medical model of psilocybin use

Western psychedelic movement, 66

White Albino (*Psilocybe cubensis* strain), 28

Whole Person, Treat the (naturopathic tenet), 163–164

Wilson, Bill, 44–45

Winkelman, Michael, 55

witches, 61–62

Wohlleben, Peter, 24

Wolfe, Tom, 66

women, as knowledge holders, 56, 58, 75

Women and Knowledge in Mesoamerica (Martinez-Cruz), 56, 75

Wound Swimming (Griego), 110

X

Xochipilli, 56, 57